Politics, Science, and Cancer: The Laetrile Phenomenon

AAAS Selected Symposia Series

 Published by Westview Press, Inc.
5500 Central Avenue, Boulder, Colorado

for the

 American Association for the Advancement of Science
1776 Massachusetts Avenue, N.W., Washington, D.C.

Politics, Science, and Cancer: The Laetrile Phenomenon

*Edited by Gerald E. Markle
and James C. Petersen*

AAAS Selected Symposium **46**

AAAS Selected Symposia Series

This book is based on a symposium which was held at the 1979 AAAS National
Annual Meeting in Houston, Texas, January 3-8. The symposium was sponsored
by the AAAS Committee on Science, Engineering, and Public Policy and by
AAAS Section K (Social and Economic Sciences).

Published in 1980 in the United States of America by
  Westview Press, Inc.
  5500 Central Avenue
  Boulder, Colorado 80301
  Frederick A. Praeger, Publisher

Library of Congress Cataloging in Publication Data
Main entry under title:
Politics, science, and cancer: the laetrile phenomenon
  (AAAS selected symposium ; v. 46)
  "Based on a symposium which was held at the 1979 AAAS National Annual
Meeting in Houston, Texas, January 3-8."
  Includes bibliographical references and index.
  1. Cancer--Chemotherapy--Social aspects--Congresses. 2. Laetrile--
Congresses. 3. Medical policy--United States--Congresses. 4. Cancer--
Law and legislation--United States--Congresses. I. Markle, Gerald E.,
1942-   II. Petersen, James C. III. American Association for the Advance-
ment of Science. IV. Series: American Association for the Advancement
of Science. AAAS selected symposium ; v. 46. (DNLM: 1. Amygdalin--Con-
gresses. 2. Legislation, Drug--United States--Congresses. 3. Public
policy--United States--Congresses.
W3 A101S v. 46 / QZ267 P769 1979)
RC271.L3P64   363.1'94   80-13466
ISBN 0-89158-854-X
ISBN 0-86531-046-7 pbk.

About the Book

At no time in U.S. history has there been a more effective challenge to medical expertise and authority than that mounted by the contemporary Laetrile movement. The efficacy of Laetrile has been debated for over twenty-five years, but despite vigorous opposition from the medical community, support for the purported cancer treatment continues to grow and the controversy has in recent years intensified and become highly politicized. How does one account for the continuing debate and the spectacular political growth of the movement to promote Laetrile? This and related questions are addressed by an interdisciplinary group of authors in this first scholarly analysis of the Laetrile phenomenon.

About the Series

The *AAAS Selected Symposia Series* was begun in 1977 to provide a means for more permanently recording and more widely disseminating some of the valuable material which is discussed at the AAAS Annual National Meetings. The volumes in this *Series* are based on symposia held at the Meetings which address topics of current and continuing significance, both within and among the sciences, and in the areas in which science and technology impact on public policy. The *Series* format is designed to provide for rapid dissemination of information, so the papers are not typeset but are reproduced directly from the camera-copy submitted by the authors. The papers are organized and edited by the symposium arrangers who then become the editors of the various volumes. Most papers published in this *Series* are original contributions which have not been previously published, although in some cases additional papers from other sources have been added by an editor to provide a more comprehensive view of a particular topic. Symposia may be reports of new research or reviews of established work, particularly work of an interdisciplinary nature, since the AAAS Annual Meetings typically embrace the full range of the sciences and their societal implications.

WILLIAM D. CAREY
Executive Officer
American Association for
the Advancement of Science

Contents

About the Editors and Authors................... xi

Acknowledgments................................ xv

1   The Laetrile Phenomenon: An Overview--
    James C. Petersen and Gerald E. Markle 1

    Actors in the Controversy   2
    Issues in the Controversy   5
    Current State of the Controversy   8
    References and Notes   8

2   Laetrile in Historical Perspective--
    James Harvey Young 11

    The Creation by the Krebs   11
    The McNaughton Ascendancy   17
    The Appeal to Freedom   24
    The Pattern of Cancer
      Unorthodoxies   38
      Exploitation of Fear,41; Promise
      of Painless Treatment and Good Results,
      42; Claims of a Miraculous Scientific
      Breakthrough,42; One Cause/One
      Therapeutic System,42; The Galileo
      Ploy,44; The Conspiracy Theory,44;
      Shifts to Adjust to Circumstances,44;
      Reliance on Testimonials,45; Distortion
      of the Idea of "Freedom,"47; Large Sums
      of Money Are Involved,47
    Laetrile Within the Perspective
      of the Past   48
    References and Notes   51

3   Laetrile at Sloan-Kettering: A Case
     Study --*Richard D. Smith* 61

4   The Political Implications of Laetrile:
     Who Gets What, When and How--*Robert F. Rich* 73

     Model of Analysis   75
     Political Background/History   76
     Competing Sets of Problem
        Definitions   76
     Definition I. Laetrile as a
        Scientific Controversy   77
        Action Implications,78
     Definition II. Laetrile as a
        Quack Cure   79
        Action Implications,80
     Definition III. Freedom of
        Choice   80
        Action Implications,82
     Definition IV. Big Government
        Interference   83
        Action Implications,83
     The Debate Over Laetrile   84
     The State Level   84
        The Legislation,84; The Role of
        the FDA,85; Other Testimony,86;
        The Role of Government,86
     Legalizing the Sale of Laetrile--
        The Implementation Phase   87
        State I,87; State II,88; State
        III,88
     The Legislative Response   89
     The Federal Level   90
     The Current Legal Status of
        Laetrile   92
        Legal Issues,92; Political Issues,93
     Discussion/Conclusions   93
        What Was at Stake? 93; Which
        Problem Definition Prevailed? 94;
        Accountability and Responsibility,
        94; "Passing the Buck,"95
     References and Notes   96

5   The Laetrile Phenomenon: Legal Perspective--
     Grace Powers Monaco 99

     Federal Drug Regulation   101
        The Regulatory Plan,101; Laetrile
        and Federal Enforcement Actions,104;

Interplay of Federal and State Statutes,112

The Informed Consent and
  Physician Liability Issues   113
The Right of Privacy   116
Physicians' Rights: The
  Privitera Case   120
Legal Implication for Cancer
  Patients   123
References and Notes   128

6   When Liberty Meets Authority: Ethical
    Aspects of the Laetrile Controversy --
    Arthur L. Caplan 133

    Should the Ethical Issues in the
      Laetrile Dispute Be Taken
      Seriously?   133
    Who Needs Government
      Regulations?   136
    Harm, Paternalism, and
      Protectionism   139
    Freedom and Paternalism   142
    Filling in the Gaps in the
      Laetrile Debate   145
    Notes   148

7   Social Context of the Laetrile Phenomenon --
    Gerald E. Markle and James C. Petersen 151

    Scientific Factors   153
    Contextual Factors   159
    Situational Factors   163
    Conclusion   168
    References and Notes   169

8   Discussion: Bias in Analysis of the
    Laetrile Controversy--*Allan Mazur* 175

9   Discussion: Science and Technology in
    the Pits--*Dorothy Nelkin* 181

Index 185

About the Editors and Authors

Gerald E. Markle, *an associate professor in the Department of Sociology at Western Michigan University, was trained in the natural sciences and the social sciences. His specific area of specialization is the sociology of science and technology and he has written about the social aspects of various cancer controversies, the ambiguities involved in the continued use of cigarettes, and the social problems involved in any widespread use of infant sex preselection techniques.*

James C. Petersen *is assistant professor of sociology and associate director of the Center for Sociological Research at Western Michigan University. A specialist in medical and political sociology and in the sociology of organizations and social movements, he has written on the topics of social participation, organizational behavior, and participant behaviors in controversies such as that surrounding Laetrile. He is currently deputy editor of the* Journal of Voluntary Action Research.

Arthur L. Caplan *is associate for the humanities, the Hastings Center, and associate for social medicine, Columbia University. A philosopher of science, he is primarily concerned with medical ethics and has written on a number of controversial issues, including medical fallibility and malpractice and aspects of the sociobiology debate. He is currently at work on* The Concepts of Health and Disease in Medicine *(Addison-Wesley, forthcoming).*

Allan Mazur, *a professor of sociology at Syracuse University, was trained in both the physical and social sciences and has made biosociology and the sociology of science and technology his two specialties. He served on the Task Force of the Presidential Advisory Group on Anticipated Advances in Science and Technology (1976) and since*

*then has served on the Biosocial Science Committee of the
Social Science Research Council. He has published numerous
articles on sociological aspects of the technological
controversies and is currently a member of the editorial
board of* Sociological Quarterly.

Grace Powers Monaco, *a partner in the law firm of
Fairman, Frisk & Monaco in Washington, D.C., specializes in
health and energy law. She represented the American Cancer
Society as amicus curiae in* United States v. Rutherford,
*the Laetrile proceeding heard by the Supreme Court in 1979.
She is a former member of the Cancer Control and Rehabilita-
tion Advisory Committee of the National Cancer Institute
and is currently president of the Candlelighters Foundation.
In 1978 she received the Annual National Award of the American Cancer Society.*

Dorothy Nelkin *is a professor in the Science, Technology
and Society Program at Cornell University. She is the author
of numerous publications on science and society, among them*
Controversy: The Politics of Technical Decisions *(Sage, 1979)
and* Science Textbook Controversies and the Politics of Equal
Time *(MIT Press, 1978). She is currently president of the
Society for the Social Studies of Science.*

Robert F. Rich *is assistant professor of politics and
public affairs in the Woodrow Wilson School, Princeton
University. A specialist in public policy analysis and
knowledge utilization, he has participated in seminars and
has written on the current Laetrile controversy. He is
editor of the journal* Knowledge: Creation, Diffusion,
Utilization *(Sage Publications).*

Richard D. Smith *is editor of* The Sciences, *the journal
of the New York Academy of Sciences. A former staff writer
and associate editor of the magazine, he has a special
interest in and has written numerous articles on the bio-
medical and behavioral sciences. He is a member of the
American Medical Writers Association and the National Association of Science Writers.*

James Harvey Young, *professor of history at Emory University, has specialized in American social and medical history, publishing in the field of food and drug regulation.*
The Toadstool Millionaires *and* The Medical Messiahs *(Princeton
University Press, 1961, 1967) trace the theme of health
quackery through American history. He has also written*

American Self-Dosage Medicines: An Historical Perspective
*(Coronado Press, 1974). He received the Edward Kremers
Award from the American Institute of the History of Pharmacy
(1962) and served the American Association for the History
of Medicine as Fielding H. Garrison Lecturer (1979).*

Acknowledgments

We owe a debt of gratitude to many people who helped make this book a reality. These include many colleagues at Western Michigan University. Bruce Clarke, David Chaplin, and Stanley Robin generously supported and encouraged our work. Several students including Roger Nemeth, Steven Severin, Gary Tibble, Ronald Troyer, and Yvonne Vissing have made substantial contributions to our study of the Laetrile phenomenon. Penne Ferguson's patience and skill as a typist greatly facilitated the preparation of this volume.

We also wish to thank the many people on both sides of the Laetrile controversy who have provided us with information and documents and consented to be interviewed. Finally we thank Kathryn Wolff, Managing Editor of Publications at AAAS, for her careful and intelligent editorial advice.

Politics, Science, and Cancer: The Laetrile Phenomenon

James C. Petersen, Gerald E. Markle

1. The Laetrile Phenomenon: An Overview

During the 1970s supporters of the purported cancer treatment Laetrile (1) have battled in the courts, state legislatures and mass media. Proponents claim that 3 grams of Laetrile daily, in conjunction with a special "metabolic" diet, will control or eliminate an active cancer in three weeks. Supporters also claim that eating ten raw apricot kernels per day will prevent cancer (2). Most medical experts and authorities have disputed these claims, viewing the use of Laetrile as quackery. For example, Robert Eyerly, Chairman of the Committee on Unproven Methods of Cancer Treatment of the American Cancer Society, has charged that "the use of Laetrile rather than known, effective cancer treatments, is the cruelest of all frauds" (3).

A major social movement had developed around the use of Laetrile (4, 5), and it has even become an element of popular culture. Drinks have been named after Laetrile -- the "B-17 Bomber" (a martini with an apricot kernel), -- Johnny Carson included Laetrile jokes in his monologues, and "Doonesbury" cartoonist Gary Trudeau showed his character 'Duke' planning to make a fortune by purchasing an apricot farm and marketing the pits in Tijuana. The movement to promote Laetrile also made impressive political and legal gains in the seventies despite opposition from the Food and Drug Administration, the American Cancer Society, the American Medical Association, and virtually the entire American medical community. In the fall of 1976 Alaska became the first state to legalize Laetrile. A 1977 Harris Poll revealed that two-thirds of all Americans favored the enactment of pro-Laetrile legislation in their state. By the summer of 1979, a total of twenty-one states had enacted such legislation (6).

Actors in the Controversy

At the core of the Laetrile movement are a few small organizations devoted to the promotion of Laetrile. The oldest of these groups, the International Association of Cancer Victims and Friends, was founded in 1963 by a woman who believed that Laetrile had cured her of cancer. The group has grown to include about 8,000 members and now promotes many alternative treatments for cancer along with Laetrile in its publication the Cancer News Journal. Schisms within this organization have spawned several new organizations that advocate holistic approaches to the treatment of cancer. These include the Cancer Control Society, a major advocate of Laetrile, as well as the Foundation for Alternative Cancer Therapies and the Cancer Federation.

The Cancer Control Society, founded by Betty Lee Morales, promotes Laetrile along with nutritional and "nontoxic" approaches to cancer therapy. It publishes the Cancer Control Journal and sponsors conventions and symposia. Among the frequent speakers at these meetings are Ernst Krebs, Jr., the discoverer of Laetrile; Dean Burk, a scientist who retired from the National Cancer Institute (NCI); and Edward Griffin, author and publicist of Laetrile.

The most influential of the pro-Laetrile organizations is, however, The Committee for Freedom of Choice in Cancer Therapy. Founded in 1972 to aid Dr. John Richardson, a California M.D. being tried for using Laetrile in cancer therapy, the Committee has grown to include over 500 local chapters. It publishes the Choice and has been extremely active in lobbying for state legislation to legalize Laetrile. The Committee has strong ties to the John Birch Society and seems to have drawn on the political experiences of this group in organizing its campaign to promote legalization of Laetrile.

The National Health Federation, an older (founded in 1955) organization concerned with health food, nutrition, and health, has also been active in the promotion of Laetrile. It established a "Fund to Stop Government Ban of Laetrile" and a newspaper, Public Scrutiny, devoted to Laetrile and metabolic therapy. Other organizations, drawn from both the political right and left, have played a peripheral role in the Laetrile movement. For example, in Wisconsin it was charged that an ultra-right group called the Posse Comitatus was linked to the manufacture of Laetrile (7). A leftist group called Second Opinion, claiming to represent the rank-and-file employees of Memorial Sloan-Kettering Cancer Center, published a report, "Laetrile at Sloan-Kettering" (8). The

report claimed that positive results with Laetrile had been
ignored and that data had been misinterpreted to make Laetrile look ineffective in laboratory studies.

All of these organizations along with other local and
regional groups have contributed to the Laetrile movement.
Many of the organizations seem to be loosely linked to one
another. Some leaders serve as officers of more than one
group and many of the same speakers turn up at conventions
and meetings of the various pro-Laetrile organizations.

We are only beginning to gain an understanding of those
individuals who advocate or actually take Laetrile. Further,
our knowledge at present is almost entirely limited to individuals with ties to the pro-Laetrile organizations. In a
study of 252 people who attended a Laetrile symposium sponsored by The Cancer Control Society (9) we found that those
attending were predominantly white, female, rural and highly
educated.   One-third of the participants belonged to pro-
Laetrile groups and almost one-half reported that they
regularly took some form of Laetrile. Comparing participants
with one another, those with higher levels of fear of cancer
were less likely to take Laetrile or to attend meetings of
Laetrile organizations. Rather than fear of cancer leading
to Laetrile use, we suspect that the causal direction is
reversed. Those who take Laetrile or are involved in the
movement are somewhat more likely to take vitamins regularly,
believe that vitamins aid in disease prevention, patronize
health food stores, and disapprove of the fluoridation of
public water. It was also found that symposium participants
were nearly ten times more likely to visit chiropractors than
are Americans generally. Furthermore, those participants
who were taking Laetrile held more positive views of the
effectiveness of chiropractors in both the prevention and
the treatment of disease than they did of M.D.s, thus
demonstrating a substantial rejection of orthodox medicine
(10).

All of these findings point toward a consistent and
connected set of ideas behind the use of Laetrile: belief
in the overriding importance of nutrition, opposition to
orthodox medicine and acceptance of officially condemned
health beliefs. Though the leaders of the Laetrile movement
often have right-wing connections, the followers seem to be
less involved with politics and more involved with health
and organic food issues. While the Laetrile controversy
has different historical roots than the health food movement,
there is clearly an overlap in membership. In fact, Laetrile advocates frequently claim that Laetrile is Vitamin B-
17 and often combine the use of Laetrile with special diets

in "nutritional" or "metabolic" therapy.

To elaborate these findings, one of our students conducted a six-month-long observation of a local chapter of the Cancer Control Society including in-depth interviews with 27 participants in the Laetrile movement (11). Twelve of these participants were taking Laetrile to treat cancer, five others were taking Laetrile as a cancer preventive, and -- interestingly -- over a third of the respondents did not take Laetrile personally although they were active in promoting its use and legalization. Respondents were highly educated and well informed about both sides of the Laetrile controversy. While they disagreed with their physicians about Laetrile, preventive medicine, and a holistic approach to treatment, they did not hold completely negative views of M.D.s or report completely negative experiences with their personal physicians. The respondents did, however, want to be able to exercise control over their lives, including medical matters. The study concluded that people become involved in the Laetrile movement more as a result of health and nutritional concerns than because of any particular experience with cancer or because of a unique political ideology.

The opposition to Laetrile has come from a prestigious coalition composed of federal agencies, the American Cancer Society, the American Medical Association, state agencies and medical societies, and medical researchers. The most visible opponent of Laetrile has been the Food and Drug Administration which has attempted to ban interstate commerce of Laetrile. As early as 1960 the FDA began to seize Laetrile and has continued such seizures to the present. The position of the FDA was most clearly stated in the "Commissioner's Decision on Status in 1977," which concluded that Laetrile is neither safe nor effective in the treatment of cancer. Thus its distribution "in interstate commerce is in violation of the Federal Food, Drug and Cosmetic Act and subject to regulatory action" (12, p. 39806).

Other federal agencies, especially the National Cancer Institute, have also been active opponents of the use of Laetrile in cancer therapy. NCI sponsored a series of tests of Laetrile in a variety of animal tumor systems. The results of these tests were uniformly negative; Laetrile showed no significant antitumor effect. In 1976 a spokesman for NCI stated:

> ...We do not at present believe there is any
> basis for the allegations made by those who
> speak publicly for Laetrile. The National

Cancer Institute certainly has not ignored
Laetrile. After extensive study, there is
in our view, no sound basis for recommending clinical trials of Laetrile (13).

However, by 1978, despite years of opposition to Laetrile,
NCI petitioned the FDA for permission to conduct clinical
trials of Laetrile. This remarkable reversal of position
was partially due to the results of a retrospective study
conducted by NCI (14), but it seems clear that social and
political pressures were important in producing the change.
Guy Newell, Deputy Director of NCI, told us:

It was thought that we would handle Laetrile
like we would any other compound in our decision network flow chart. You see it is not
a matter of all or none. We have a battery
of compounds to go through animal testing.
And it really is a matter of prioritizing.
Laetrile is on the list somewhere but we have
other compounds that have shown up so much
better and we have only limited human clinical resources so we pick higher priority
drugs. We never would have gotten down to
Laetrile. So Laetrile was really taken out
of priority...and I think not for scientific
reasons. I think because of other reasons:
social, political, human (15).

Several private organizations have been vigorous opponents of the Laetrile movement. Both the American Medical
Association and the American Cancer Society have labeled the
use of Laetrile in the treatment of cancer as quackery. ACS
has been especially active in distributing literature attacking the use of Laetrile. Memorial Sloan-Kettering Cancer
Center has also made well-publicized attacks on Laetrile,
claiming that a series of animal studies conducted by Sloan-
Kettering showed no anti-cancer effects.

Issues in the Controversy

The Laetrile controversy is in fact composed of several
interrelated disputes. At issue are both knowledge factors
where scientific claims are made and rebutted and value
factors where philosophical, political, and constitutional
issues are debated.

The central knowledge claim of Laetrile proponents is
that cancer is not a tumor disease; instead it is a metabolic disease in which the tumor is merely an obvious

symptom. In this view cancer arises from trophoblasts which
are primitive, undifferentiated cells which survive early
pregnancy. First formulated by John Beard in 1902 and re-
fined by Ernst Krebs, Jr. in the 1940s and 1950s, the
"unitarian" or trophoblastic theory rejects the notion that
cancer is caused by unnatural invasion; rather the disease
results from uncontrolled trophoblastic growth. As the
theory was elaborated by Krebs and others, a biochemical
mechanism was proposed by which Laetrile destroyed cancerous
growths. Cancer cells, the advocates claimed, have excessive
amounts of an enzyme which frees cyanide from the complex
Laetrile molecule. The cyanide thus selectively poisons
cancer cells while leaving healthy cells alone. More recently, Laetrile proponents have attempted to incorporate
the idea that Laetrile is a vitamin (B-17) into these
theories. Most cancer researchers reject the trophoblastic
thesis. Medical experts also dispute the various claims
made for the biochemical mechanisms proposed for Laetrile
(12, pp. 39773-39775).

Critics of Laetrile have asserted that the use of
Laetrile is not only ineffective but actually dangerous.
Several deaths have been attributed to Laetrile poisoning.
In one such case in 1977, a 10-month-old girl died, purportedly after swallowing five of her father's 500 mg. Laetrile
tablets. The medical examiner attributed her death to
"excessive anoxic brain damage due to acute cyanide poisoning due to amygdalin ingestion" (16). Laetrile advocates
counter these claims with epidemiological data. Most often
cited are the Hunzakuts, a remote Pakistani tribe. Apparently it is not uncommon for these people to live 100 years,
and their longevity is attributed to a diet rich in amygdalin. In addition it is claimed that cancer is absent
among these people, although a 1955 Japanese expedition did
report incidence of the dread disease (17). The current
view at the National Cancer Institute is that oral ingestion
of Laetrile is more dangerous than Laetrile injections. In
fact NCI proposes to use both intravenous injections and oral
administration in its proposed clinical trial of Laetrile.

Theory aside, the most important claim made for Laetrile
is that it saves lives. Only one pro-Laetrile clinical study
has been published in an American medical journal. Reporting on patients treated with Laetrile the author concluded
that: "possible regression of the malignant lesion was
suggested by therapeutic results in 10 cases of inoperable
cancer with metastases" (18). Studies from Germany and the
Philippines also claim that Laetrile is efficacious. The
most elaborate and dramatic claims for Laetrile have been
made by John A. Richardson in his book Laetrile Case

Histories, published by Bantam Books in 1977. The FDA Commissioner has sharply criticized Richardson's work, claiming
that he reported only 62 of some 4,000 case studies and that
patient follow-ups were irregular (12, p. 39778).

In response to the claims of Laetrile advocates, NCI
sponsored laboratory research on mouse tumors at Arthur D.
Little, Inc., the Southern Research Institute, Washington
University, Battelle Memorial Institute, and Memorial Sloan-
Kettering Cancer Center. In each of these studies Laetrile
was found to be inactive against a variety of tumor systems,
although considerable controversy arose from charges of am-
biguous findings and deceit at Sloan-Kettering. Moreover,
in 1977 a Loyola biologist claimed that Laetrile, as part of
a megavitamin regimen, effectively controlled mammary tumors
in mice (19). Despite the fact that the paper was presented
in a non-scholarly setting, that the paper was only two pages
long, and that the experimental design lacked certain controls, the paper received national media attention.

While empirical issues and knowledge claims have and
will continue to shape the Laetrile controversy, an equal
role has been played by value disputes. Some political philosophers, particularly conservative ones, have joined with
health advocates and Laetrile proponents in asserting that
personal and constitutional freedom are the real issues of
the controversy. Cancer patients, they declare, have a
right to choose their own form of cancer therapy without
interference from the medical community or the government.
This issue, referred to as "freedom of choice," has been the
single most effective argument that Laetrile proponents have
used in the courts, state legislatures and media.

Medical authorities, particularly the FDA, contend that
freedom of choice is a slogan used to promote a cynical and
cruel hoax. They claim that government must prevent deception and the victimization of the weak. They also claim
that cancer patients and their families, because of the
severe emotional trauma of the disease, are incapable of
choosing freely. Rather they should rely on qualified experts to advise them. This debate, though part of Laetrile's
history, clearly transcends the fate of any one purported
cancer cure.

Laetrile proponents have not only asserted the right to
make key medical decisions, they have stressed the desir-
ability of such actions. In a number of important ways they
are connected with the holistic health movement. Advocates
of Laetrile frequently call for a rejection of medical expertise and a deprofessionalization of medical care. They

emphasize the individual's responsibility for his or her own health and the need for concern with the prevention of cancer.

Current State of the Controversy

The dispute over Laetrile remains in flux. With the Rutherford and other cases still being adjudicated, with the NCI attempting to begin clinical trials, and with state legislatures still considering the deregulation of Laetrile, it is premature to predict the future direction of the controversy (20). Given the momentum of the controversy as well as its complexity, it seems likely that Laetrile will retain its prominence in our culture for some time.

On June 18, 1979, the U.S. Supreme Court unanimously upheld the FDA's authority to ban the distribution of Laetrile to terminally ill cancer patients. The 10th Circuit Court of Appeals, the Supreme Court ruled, had erred in its conclusion that the "safety and effectiveness standards... could have no reasonable application to terminal patients" (21). However, the court did not rule on several broad constitutional issues, but rather remanded the case back to the Appeals Court for further consideration. Further litigation, perhaps lasting years, seems likely.

The safety and effectiveness of Laetrile is also likely to remain in doubt for years. Even if the proposed NCI trials do occur, the outcome is not likely to be definitive. The normal ambiguity of science, compounded by the distrust which has and will continue to characterize the controversy, makes speedy resolution of the controversy unlikely.

References and Notes

1.   Laetrile is also known as amygdalin and Vitamin B-17.
     However it now appears that amygdalin, a substance found
     naturally in the seeds and kernels of many fruits (most
     notably apricots) and grains is not identical to Laet-
     rile. Moreover, FDA Commissioner Donald Kennedy charges
     that confusion over the terms may be a deliberate effort
     by promoters to obfuscate the efficacy issue (Federal
     Register 42, 39771, 1977). Authorities also deny that
     Laetrile is a vitamin. According to the American Insti-
     tute of Nutrition, there is "no scientific evidence that
     Laetrile has nutrient properties or is in any way of
     nutritional value for either animals or humans" (Journal
     of the American Medical Association, 236, 1284, 1976).
2.   McNaughton Foundation, Physician's Handbook of Vitamin

B-17 Therapy (Science Press International, Sausalito, 1973).

3. R. Eyerly, "Laetrile: Focus on the Facts," CA 26, 50-54, (1976).

4. J. C. Petersen and G. E. Markle, "The Laetrile Controversy," in Controversy: Politics of Technical Decisions, D. Nelkin, ed. (Sage, Beverly Hills, 1979).

5. J. C. Petersen and G. E. Markle, "Politics and Science in the Laetrile Controversy," Social Studies of Science 9, forthcoming (1979).

6. The twenty-one states are: Alaska, Arizona, Colorado, Delaware, Florida, Idaho, Illinois, Indiana, Kansas, Louisiana, Maryland, Montana, Nevada, New Hampshire, New Jersey, North Dakota, Oklahoma, Oregon, South Dakota, Texas, and Washington. Tennessee

7. N. D. Rosenberg, "Right Wing Group Tied to Laetrile," Milwaukee Journal (22 May 1977).

8. Second Opinion, Laetrile at Sloan-Kettering: Second Opinion Special Report (Second Opinion, New York, 1977).

9. G. E. Markle, J. C. Petersen, and M. O. Wagenfeld, "Notes from the Cancer Underground: Participation in the Laetrile Movement," Social Science and Medicine 12, 31-37 (1978).

10. M. O. Wagenfeld, Y. Vissing, G. E. Markle, and J. C. Petersen, "Notes from the Cancer Underground: Health Attitudes and Practices of Participants in the Laetrile Movement," Social Science and Medicine, forthcoming, 1979.

11. Y. M. Vissing, "An Exploratory Analysis of Participation in the Laetrile Movement," unpublished M.A. thesis, Western Michigan University, 1978.

12. D. Kennedy, "Laetrile: Commissioner's Decision on Status," Federal Register 42 (151), 39768-39806 (1977).

13. R. J. Avery, Office of Cancer Communication, National Cancer Institute, personal communication (4 March 1976).

14. N. E. Ellison, D. P. Byar, and G. R. Newell, "Results of the National Cancer Institute's Retrospective Laetrile Analysis," New England Journal of Medicine 299, 549-552 (1978).

15. Interview with G. R. Newell (8 March 1979).

16. Cited in J. F. Ross, "The Harmful Effects of Laetrile, Apricot Kernel and Cyanogenic Fruit and Vegetable Materials on Human Beings; and the Ineffectiveness of Laetrile as a Therapeutic Agent in Patients With Cancer," Statement to the U.S. Subcommittee on Health and Scientific Research (12 July 1977), 66.

17. N. Harada and A. Miyoshi, "Is the 'Healthy Hunza' True?" in Personality and Health in Hunza Valley, K. Imanishi, ed. (Kyoto University, Kyoto, 1963).

18. J. A. Morrone, "Chemotherapy of Inoperable Cancer: Pre-
    liminary Report of 10 Cases Treated With Laetrile,"
    Experimental Medicine and Surgery 20, 299-308 (1962).
19. H. W. Manner, "The Remission of Tumors With Laetrile,"
    paper presented before the meetings of the National
    Health Federation, 1978.
20. G. E. Markle and J. C. Petersen, "Resolution of the
    Laetrile Controversy: Past Attempts and Future Pros-
    pects," paper presented at a session in the project,
    Elements and Principles of Closure in Ethical and
    Scientific Disputes, The Hastings Center, 16 June 1979.
21. United States v. G. Rutherford, Supreme Court of the
    United States, No. 78-605 (18 June 1979).

2. Laetrile in Historical Perspective

Laetrile's history has been complex, tortuous, kaleido-scopic. Beginning inauspiciously like hundreds of other small-time anti-cancer schemes, Laetrile soared to a notori-ous pinnacle as the unorthodox brand-name health promotion generating the largest amount of public furor in the nation's history. Numerous actors played roles in this perfervid drama. Laetrile's history, first, may be placed within three successive periods which may be designated: the creation by the Krebs, the McNaughton ascendancy, the appeal to freedom. Then the Laetrile pattern may be compared with the pattern of earlier cancer unorthodoxies.

The Creation by the Krebs

Two men, each named Ernst T. Krebs, father and son, bring Laetrile to market and dominate its early years. Their backgrounds may prove instructive.

Ernst Krebs, Sr., born in 1876, son of a California pharmacist, himself worked as a pharmacist before attending the San Francisco College of Physicians and Surgeons (1,2). He received his medical degree in 1903. Practicing in Nevada during the influenza pandemic of 1918, Dr. Krebs became persuaded that an old Indian remedy possessed great efficacy in combatting the flu. A rare species of parsley, Leptotoemia dissecta, Krebs wrote in a Nevada State Board of Health bulletin, had permitted the Washoe Indians to survive the epidemic without loss of life, whereas members of other tribes died in great numbers (3,4).

Krebs promptly commercialized his discovery. In San Francisco he set up the Balsamea Company to market a pro-prietary named Syrup Leptinol, recommended for use in epidemic influenza, bronchial asthma, whooping cough,

pneumonia, and pulmonary tuberculosis (5). A later version
called Syrup Bal-Sa-Me-A, with rhubarb added, bore labeling
which recounted how Leptotoemia had protected the Washoes and
which promised users "miraculous results" (6). "It strikes
at the cause," the circular read, "quickly checking germ
action." Such claims so disturbed Krebs' fellow physicians
that he resigned from medical societies and never rejoined
(1). Such claims also disturbed the Bureau of Chemistry of
the Department of Agriculture, in charge of enforcing the
Pure Food and Drugs Act of 1906. The Bureau had shipments
of Krebs' proprietary seized in Missouri, Illinois, and Oregon, terming its labeling false and fraudulent (5, 6). When
no claimants appeared, courts condemned the medicines and
ordered them destroyed. Dr. Krebs did not give up on his
product. At the end of the 1950s a Syrup of Balsamea was
still being sold, and Krebs' promotion contained the suggestion that he had discovered the first antibiotic (7, 8). No
longer an over-the-counter proprietary, Krebs now distributed
Balsamea under the guise of an investigational prescription
drug.

In the intervening years Dr. Krebs had continued to seek
new therapeutic entities. Before 1951, when Laetrile surfaced surely in the public record, he had been involved with
both cancer treatments and apricot kernels. Krebs had promoted an enzyme, chymotrypsin, as a cancer remedy, explaining
its action by the same trophoblastic theory, borrowed from
John Beard, a turn-of-the-century Edinburgh embryologist,
that was to undergird later Laetrile promotion (9). And in
1945 Krebs submitted a New Drug Application (NDA) for a drug
called Allergenase, manufactured from the kernels of shelled
apricot seeds, and claimed to be "a systemic detoxicant" for
treating all allergies, including arthritis, asthma, and
"shingles" (10, 11). He had begun work on this drug, he said,
in 1924. In due course Allergenase evolved into pangamic
acid, otherwise known as Vitamin B-15.

Dr. Krebs told two tales about Laetrile's origin. The
earlier account ascribed a recent discovery date. The later
account, furnished in a court affidavit signed by Dr. Krebs
in 1965, provided a more remote origin. As of 1965, having
a long history for Laetrile had become legally important,
because of so-called "grandfather" clauses relating to drugs
in both the 1938 Food, Drug, and Cosmetic Act and the 1962
Kefauver-Harris Amendments to that law. Drugs in use before
critical dates escaped some aspects of regulation.

Some versions of the Laetrile legend traced the drug's
origin to Dr. Krebs' researches in the 1920s aimed at making
bootleg liquor palatable (12). In his 1965 affidavit Krebs

stated that he had first made an extract from apricot kernels in 1926, calling it Sarcarcinase, containing amygdalin, a chemical known for a century (13). A later critic has denied that Sarcarcinase could have been Laetrile's amygdalin-containing ancestor, because Sarcarcinase was a chloroform extract of apricot kernels, and the amygdalin would have gone down the drain with the discarded aqueous portion (14). In any case, Dr. Krebs stated in his affidavit that Sarcarcinase proved too toxic a drug when injected into rats. Steadily improving his extraction process, Krebs asserted, he achieved an ever higher level of amygdalin purity. In 1949 Krebs' son slightly modified his father's process and named the result Laetrile. This version of Laetrile's origin became the standard canon among its promoters.

The earlier tale that Dr. Krebs had told about Laetrile's beginning dated its birth to 1951. In an interview with Food and Drug Administration officials during December 1952, Dr. Krebs said that ten months before he had begun experimenting with a cyanogenetic glucoside which he had extracted from a mixture containing apricot pits (15). He had tested it successfully on patients, he asserted, but had kept no records. Injected near the site of a cancerous lesion, Laetrile worked by liquefying the malignant growth through the release of cyanide.

Soon Dr. Krebs and his son presented a more elaborate explanation for Laetrile's mode of action. The theory proved to be the same one which they had recently used to justify the presumed anti-cancer activity of an enzyme with which they had been experimenting.

Ernst Krebs, Jr., who coined the name Laetrile, had come home to California after peripatetic schooling. He did not have a Ph.D. from the University of Illnois, as he sometimes asserted, nor had he yet received his only claim to the doctorate, an honorary Doctor of Science degree from the American Christian College in Tulsa, Oklahoma (16). According to California state investigators, Krebs had attended colleges in Mississippi, Tennessee, and California before receiving a bachelor of arts degree in 1942 from the University of Illinois. Also before going to Illinois, Krebs had spent three years as a medical student at Hahnemann Medical College in Philadelphia, the second of which was a repetition of the first year's work. Krebs devoted two years, from 1943 to 1945, to graduate study of anatomy at the University of California, but was dismissed because of his pursuit of what was deemed unorthodoxy (17).

Krebs, Jr., continued his researches in collaboration

with Dr. Charles Gurchot, a pharmacologist who also had left
the university (18). The two had published a letter in Science, "Growth of Trophoblast in the Anterior Chamber of the
Eye of the Rabbit" (19), and now set up a foundation bearing
Beard's name to seek a cancer cure fitting his principles (18).

In 1950 Krebs-pere and -fils published their own version
of Beard's trophoblastic or unitarian thesis (9). All
cancer, they asserted, is one, brought on when the normal
trophoblast cell goes wrong. This cell, which in both sexes
emerges from a very primitive cell, is best known for its
role in securing the embryo to the uterine wall. This function, the Krebs stated, demands erosion, infiltration, and
metastasizing. In becoming cancerous, trophoblasts do the
same things, dangerously. Beard had said that some pancre-
atic enzymes attack trophoblasts. The Krebs and Gurchot
had found an enzyme they believed to be specifically antithetical to malignant cells.

The 1950 article, seeing great promise in the enzyme
chymotrypsin, did not mention Laetrile. At about the very
same time, however, -- at least, according to Dr. Krebs'
1952 account -- Laetrile was born. And soon the Krebs presented a Beardian explanation for Laetrile's mode of action.
The Laetrile molecule, the theory held, when it reached the
site of the cancer, was hydrolyzed by an enzyme, beta-
glucosidase, releasing cancer-killing hydrogen cyanide (20,
21). This enzyme accumulated in cancerous areas in much
greater quantity than it did in healthy cells, so the cyanide was released where it was needed. Moreover, normal
cells were protected by another enzyme, rhodanese, which
detoxified any cyanide that might be liberated in or stray
to them. Cancerous cells lacked rhodanese. Thus Laetrile,
according to its promoters' theory, fulfilled a prime objective of the nascent field of cancer chemotherapy, speci-
ficity of action: it targeted damage to cancerous cells
without injuring normal cells unduly.

Right from the start Laetrile became related to a
number of separate but intertwining organizations, legally
distinct but linked, at least so FDA officials came to
believe, through Ernst Krebs, Jr., their "guiding light"
(8, 22). The John Beard Memorial Foundation, the research
unit, became Krebs, Sr.'s province. Krebs, Jr., personally
supervised production in the Krebs' Research Laboratories.
The finished product then went to the Spicer-Gerhart Company
in Pasadena which distributed Laetrile as an investigational
drug. Some California general practitioners began to use it
in treating patients with cancer, and requests for it came
in from other states and from overseas. A New Jersey group

of doctors, for example, used Laetrile. Their business
manager, Glenn Kittler, upon hearing a tape recording of
Krebs' explanation of the trophoblastic theory, responded
by opining that Krebs was "well on his way toward the Nobel
Prize" (22).

California cancer specialists were not so quickly persuaded. The Cancer Commission of the California Medical
Association sought to secure some Laetrile from Krebs to
permit a clinical trial under the direction of the Research
Committee and the Tumor Board of the Los Angeles Hospital.
While "anxious" to have clinical work commenced, Krebs, Jr.,
replied, he foresaw difficulties (23). Especially he ob-
jected to tests made by physicians ignorant of trophoblastic
theory. "Conducting work under these conditions," he wrote,
"is almost tantamount to attempting to conduct an orderly
practical industrial implementation of nuclear fission with
the cooperation of physicists who failed to accept the $E=mc^2$
formula and were gravely in doubt about the atomic constitution of matter." Unless a doctor of his own choosing could
direct the experiment, Krebs would send no Laetrile. Such
a stance recurred not infrequently in Laetrile's future: an
expressed desire, sometimes a demand, for trials, but heel-
dragging about complying with the established parameters of
scientific research, a denial that mainstream scientists
could test Laetrile fairly. In Krebs' metaphor from physics,
be it noted, he baldly transposed orthodoxy and unorthodoxy.

With a supply of Laetrile secured from the Food and
Drug Administration (24), the Cancer Commission of the California Medical Association sponsored at three cancer research centers controlled trials of Laetrile as a treatment
for various cancers in mice (25). None of the tests revealed that Laetrile had any effect on the course of the disease.
The Commission also assembled as much information as it
could about patients who had been treated with Laetrile --
forty-four cases in all -- and found no objective evidence
that Laetrile alone exercised any control over cancer. The
conclusion was based on examination of seventeen cancer
sufferers still alive and on autopsies of nine of the nine-
teen patients who had died. Furthermore, the Commission
disputed the explanation by the Krebs as to how Laetrile
purportedly functioned. The molecule-cleaving enzyme which
supposedly released hydrogen cyanide at the site of the
cancer, held by the Krebs to be more abundant in cancerous
than in normal cells, in fact, said the Commission, was not;
normal cells contained more of the enzyme than did neoplas-
tic tissue. In time scientists were to presume that, because of the extremely small concentrations of beta-
glucosidase in human tissues, Laetrile administered

parenterally would undergo scarcely any metabolic breakdown and would leave the body in the urine virtually intact (26).

Krebs, Jr., and the small coterie of Laetrile physicians dismissed the California Cancer Commission's report. A newer improved version of Laetrile and new dosage levels, they said, invalidated the Commission's distorted findings (22, 27). In any case, asserted one Laetrile doctor, no curative claims had ever been held out, only the promise of stopping the cancer's growth and prolonging the patient's life with diminished pain and greater comfort. Despite the denial, Dr. Krebs, Sr., had in fact been quoted in the press as saying that Laetrile wrought cures in forty percent of cancer patients and brought improvement to the remaining sixty percent (28).

Laetrile's proponents no doubt welcomed controversy as a way of making their product better known. They had courted publicity. The Cancer Commission first heard about Laetrile through a barrage of inquiries from national magazines, news services, and the California press (25). A Laetrile physician had given a list of his patients to a newspaper, inviting reporters to interview and photograph them. Krebs, Jr., worked hard at expanding the market for his investigational drug. Some insight into his zeal may be derived from what he wrote, some years later, to an entrepreneur hoping to market Laetrile under his own trade name in foreign areas: ". . . [T]he field of cancer chemotherapy is a law to itself. This jungle offers the greatest opportunity anywhere in commerce at this moment, but there are snakes in every bush. I believe . . . it's best to push hard, sell, don't be backward about disaffecting a few, and establish . . . [Laetrile] right from the start as something precious that not even hospitals get for nothing" (29). In the same letter Krebs noted: ". . . [O]ne can usually buy even the top medical investigators as one does sirloin steak -- and at about the same price."

In fact, reports suggesting Laetrile's utility in cancer came not from the top but from a few clinicians overseas and several American general practitioners (26). American cancer experts dismissed the pro-Laetrile studies as purely anecdotal or so poorly designed as to lack validity. If the market grew for Laetrile during the 1950s, it was at a modest rate. Krebs, Jr., secured a British patent for the product, but it did not mention cancer (30). He joined with Fred J. Hart, a promoter of therapeutic devices, in testifying against a California bill aimed at curbing cancer quackery, but the law passed anyway (31). Another signal ominous for the Krebs appeared at the start of the new

decade. In 1960 the Food and Drug Administration made its
first seizure of an interstate shipment of Laetrile. That
same year a decade of litigation had finally driven Harry
Hoxsey from the field of cancer quackery (32). His successor
at the Dallas clinic, barred from using Hoxsey's mix of
botanicals, had ordered the lot of Laetrile which the FDA
had seized (33).

The Food and Drug Administration had watched the Laetrile venture from its early days. The California Cancer
Commission critique of 1953 raised the question of taking
regulatory steps. After weighing the matter at the highest
level, FDA opted for continuing close scrutiny of operations,
not immediate action. Other projects held higher priority,
and manpower was short. Laetrile was both small in size and
difficult to combat. ". . . [T]his type of promotion, namely
an article distributed as a new drug for investigational purposes but indirectly promoted for use in cancer, is hard to
handle" (34). So concluded a headquarters memorandum. If
Laetrile were directly offered as a cancer treatment in
printed labeling, chances for controlling it through regulation would be "brighter." Thus the Krebs' cautious approach,
depending mainly on word of mouth promotion instead of bold
labeling claims, postponed trouble, probably at the expense
of growth. The 1960 seizure signaled a change.

The first period of Laetrile's history, during which
the Krebs' brand of amygdalin, shrewdly but cautiously promoted, made modest gains without encountering serious regulatory troubles, ended about 1963. By then both state and
federal governments, the latter with powerful new weapons
given it by the Kefauver-Harris law, had attacked in force.
Public worry about drugs, cued by Senator Estes Kefauver's
hearings and the frightening thalidomide episode, which lay
behind the Tennessee Senator's law, had soared to new
heights. Besieged by regulatory actions, the Krebs yielded
real control over their enterprise to a Canadian citizen
possessing capital, audacity, and a broader vision of Laetrile's destiny.

The McNaughton Ascendancy

Andrew Robert Leslie McNaughton first met Ernst Krebs,
Jr., so McNaughton testified, in a Miami drugstore in 1956
or 1957 (35). Shortly before this, McNaughton had infor-
mally set up a foundation in Montreal, incorporated in 1958,
to support researchers possessing unorthodox but possibly
useful ideas who found it difficult to secure funds else-
where. In 1960, after spending several weeks in the Krebs'
San Francisco laboratory, McNaughton took some Laetrile back

with him to Canada, persuaded several tobacco companies to
contribute research funds, and, through his McNaughton Foundation, distributed Laetrile to a number of Quebec physicians
as an investigational drug. In 1961 McNaughton founded Biozymes International Ltd., a manufacturing concern, which the
next year began to produce Laetrile (36).

McNaughton came from a notable family and had enjoyed a
glamorous if at times checkered career (36, 37, 38). His
father had headed Canada's armed forces during World War II.
The son had served as chief test pilot for the Royal Canadian Air Force. He had sold arms to Israel and had let Fidel
Castro capture weapons which McNaughton had been commission-
ed to sell to Batista, the Cuban president, for use in
suppressing Castro's insurgency. In time McNaughton and his
foundation became targets of a suit brought by the U.S.
Securities and Exchange Commission, charging promotion and
sale of unregulated securities, stock in Biozymes International. In 1973 a district court in California, not having received an answer to the complaint, rendered a default judgment of permanent injunction (39).

Besides launching his Laetrile enterprises in Canada,
McNaughton undertook an initiative in the United States.
Taking Krebs, Jr., and a pro-Laetrile physician along,
McNaughton went to Washington. Through the good offices of
a New Jersey Congressman, he secured conferences with Health,
Education and Welfare and Food and Drug Administration officials (40, 41). What would it take, the Laetrile party
asked, to have a New Drug Application favorably considered?
Krebs explained the rationale behind Laetrile's purported
action, indicating that dosage levels now were higher than
those first used. No claims for cure of cancer would be
made, only for palliation. While safety data seemed complete, evidence of effectiveness admittedly rested on clinical research outside the nation's borders, although three
United States clinical investigations were under way. In
the granting of an NDA was only safety considered? Not,
FDA officials replied, with drugs prescribed for life-
threatening diseases. In such cases safety and efficacy
could not be separated. An innocuous product which failed
to help the patient would constitute a hazard when used in
lieu of treatment that offered some promise of success.
Without sound clinical evidence from recognized experts, the
government men told Krebs and McNaughton, a New Drug Application could not be deemed complete.

In November 1961 the FDA charged Krebs and the John
Beard Memorial Foundation with violating the law (42). The
case involved not Laetrile, but Krebs' other major product,

pangamic acid or Vitamin B-15. Krebs had shipped capsules
of this new drug into Oregon and Florida without having an
effective NDA, in the same way in which he was distributing
Laetrile. Both the Foundation and its sole officer pleaded
guilty to the charge, Krebs being fined $3750 and sentenced
to prison. Imprisonment was suspended when Krebs agreed to
the terms of a three-year probation. One of those terms
barred Krebs and his Foundation from manufacturing and distributing Laetrile until there should be an approved NDA.
The court shortly agreed to a modification of the probation
order permitting Krebs to exhaust the supply of Laetrile on
hand by shipping it without payment to the McNaughton Foundation in Montreal and to a few physicians in the United
States so that experiments might continue (43, 44). Laetrile patients and their families had written pleading
letters to the judge.

When the small reserve supply of Laetrile came to an
end, interstate distribution supposedly would cease. NDAs
submitted by both Krebs, Jr., and Krebs, Sr., fell short of
meeting FDA's standards for acceptance (45). Krebs, Jr.,
and the John Beard Memorial Foundation obeyed the court's
ruling and stopped making Laetrile. But production and distribution did not stop. Krebs, Sr., and Krebs Laboratories,
according to FDA records, picked up the task. And McNaughton's Canadian venture quickened. He got some of his raw
material for making Laetrile from England, Krebs, Jr.,
thought, and for one stage in the production process sent
the drug into New Jersey (46).

Indeed, McNaughton increasingly made his powerful presence felt on the entire Laetrile scene. He strove, without
success, to get the Damon Runyon Cancer Fund to evaluate
Laetrile, reaping some headlines from the effort (47). However, a vastly more successful publicity coup soon followed.
The American Weekly, a Hearst publication, during March 1963
ran two articles presenting Laetrile in a most favorable
light (48). They were followed shortly by a paperback book
from which they had been taken, Laetrile, Control for Cancer
(2). "The most important medical news of our time," the
cover promised, "First major breakthrough in the cancer
mystery. The day is near when no one need die from cancer.
LAETRILE, the revolutionary new anti-cancer drug . . . WILL
BE TO CANCER WHAT INSULIN IS TO DIABETES." Written by Glenn
D. Kittler, who earlier had acclaimed Krebs, Jr., as Nobel
Prize material, the book presented a highly dramatic version
of Laetrile's discovery and a most optimistic rendering of
Krebs-sponsored clinical experience with the drug. To use
the term "cures" for cancer Kittler considered "inaccurate,"
but he added: "The idea of a cancer control, on the other

hand, is perfectly plausible. In the minds of an increasing
number of leading scientists, the best control now available
is Laetrile." The book concluded by quoting Andrew McNaughton to the same effect. McNaughton contributed also the
book's foreword, to which he appended his Foundation's Montreal address. Letters of inquiry sent to the Foundation
received replies saying Laetrile might soon be available
from Canada and asking cancer sufferers to have their doctors
write the Foundation (49). Some United States citizens
crossed the border to Montreal to get Laetrile injections (50).

While thus deeply involved in a publicity venture tre-
mendously expanding Laetrile's national visibility, McNaughton also worked away on other fronts. He sent Laetrile made
in Canada to a foreign trade zone in San Francisco for trans-
shipment to markets in the Far and Middle East (51). And he
continued to deal with the Krebs. Relations were sometimes
tense, but McNaughton -- at least in the judgment of obser-
ving food and drug officials -- came to assume the upper
hand (52). In speaking of Laetrile, he often used the pro-
prietary "we," and he acted as if he were making the important decisions. When the probation stock of Laetrile ran
out, it was McNaughton who went to Washington, this time
alone, to see if he could pressure the FDA into letting him
have more, arguing that he should not be penalized for the
misdeeds of Ernst Krebs, Jr. (53). FDA officials pointed
out that Laetrile still did not have a completed NDA and
that the new Kefauver law had stiffened standards for ad-
mitting new drugs to the market.

Legal difficulties, indeed, soon cast shadows across
the publicity coup resulting from Kittler's book. California, after holding hearings under its new law aimed at
specious cancer treatments, banned Laetrile as a quack remedy (54, 55). The Canadian Food and Drug Directorate barred
further distribution of Laetrile by the McNaughton Foundation on the grounds that its safety and efficacy had not
been proved (56). McNaughton, calling unconstitutional the
law under which the Directorate had moved, sought in 1964 to
enjoin the Directorate from enforcing it. But McNaughton
lost in court. The next year the Food and Drug Administration strove to curb Dr. Krebs, Sr.'s small-scale but per-
sistent shipment of Laetrile in interstate commerce. After
protracted court action, he was enjoined, later cited for
criminal contempt, and finally fined for violating his probation (57). Dr. Krebs probably prescribed Laetrile for his
patients through the remainder of his life, although he gave
up manufacturing and distributing it, while maintaining the
production of pangamic acid (58). He died in 1970 from a
fall on the stairs at the age of 94 (59, 60).

In the meantime, Andrew McNaughton had moved to California. Both the Krebs, father and son, had been enjoined from dealing in Laetrile, and in Canada so had McNaughton himself. Using several corporate names, McNaughton continued the manufacture of Laetrile in San Francisco, then in Sausalito (38, 61), and from his transplanted McNaughton Foundation he tried once more in 1970 to get FDA approval for experimental use of Laetrile on human subjects (62, 63, 64). McNaughton's submission of an IND, an Investigational New Drug application, a document required by the Kefauver-Harris Act before human trials could proceed, became a cause célèbre. Upon receipt of the IND, the FDA routinely approved it, in accordance with then prevailing practice. A quick appraisal did not reveal in the application the kind of promising evidence from animal experimentation that would provide a reasonable basis for expecting anti-tumor activity in man. Eight days later the FDA wrote McNaughton that the IND could not be continued without more satisfactory data, and when no new information arrived before the deadline set in regulations, the FDA cancelled the application. Further information later submitted by McNaughton did not persuade Food and Drug officials to change their minds. Manufacturing controls and preclinical and clinical data all remained unsatisfactory.

Laetrile supporters reinterpreted these events into a tale of FDA's perfidy. According to this version, FDA's initial automatic acceptance of an IND until the evidence could be examined became instead a bona fide acceptance which the agency then reversed under pressure from the political moguls of the cancer research establishment (65, 66). A pro-Laetrile reporter predicted "a showdown" between the hidden forces of repressive orthodoxy and champions of alternate modalities (65).

A showdown did indeed occur. A varied constellation of circumstances had moved the Laetrile cause upward on the path of political power. Not only had Hoxsey's star set through governmental action and exposure, so too had Krebiozen's virtual demise arrived by 1966, thus creating a vacuum at the apex of cancer unorthodoxy ready for filling by a new contender. The publicity generated by Kittler's book gave Laetrile a good boost toward the top. Moreover, McNaughton gained a recruit to his cause from the inner citadel of the cancer research establishment who was destined to play for Laetrile something like the role Andrew Ivy had played for Krebiozen. Dean Burk, who had received his Ph.D. in biochemistry from the University of California, had devoted a more than forty-year career to cancer investigation, with many honors along the way, and now was chief of the Cytochemistry Section of the National Cancer Institute (65, 67). In 1968 McNaughton

had persuaded Burk to undertake research on Laetrile, and by
the time two years later of FDA's rejection of the McNaughton
Foundation's IND, Burk had become a fervent Laetrile cham-
pion, calling many of his contrary-minded governmental associates "scientifically immoral" (65). Stepped-up Laetrile
publicity focused the spotlight on Burk.

The scope of Laetrile publicity had also broadened because a new organization had sprung up to wave its banner
and because an established league of unorthodox health promoters had taken up Laetrile's cause. The new group, the
International Association of Cancer Victims and Friends, was
founded in 1963 by a San Diego schoolteacher, Cecile Pollack
Hoffman (50, 68). She herself had turned to Laetrile with
despair and hope. In 1959 she had sustained a radical mas-
tectomy because of breast cancer, and three years later the
spread of cancer led to further surgery. She learned of
Laetrile when her husband saw a copy of Kittler's book in an
airport lobby. Cued by McNaughton's foreword, Mrs. Hoffman
journeyed to Montreal for Laetrile injections. She continued receiving them closer to home, by crossing the border to
Tijuana, becoming the first Laetrile patient of a Mexican
physician, Ernesto Contreras Rodriguez. Persuaded that
Laetrile had saved her life, angry that this treatment was
not legally available in the United States, Mrs. Hoffman
established her International Association. Through print,
meetings, and personal evangelism, the association castigated
"out-of-date, out-moded, so-called 'orthodox' treatment,"
and vigorously espoused what Mrs. Hoffman termed "non-toxic,
beneficial therapies," especially Laetrile. Krebs, Jr.,
Contreras, and in time Dean Burk addressed IACVF assemblies
(69, 70, 71). The organization provided cancer sufferers
with information on how to get to Tijuana. When Canada
joined the United States in making Laetrile illegal, Dr.
Contreras' business boomed. Mrs. Hoffman died in 1969 of
metastatic cancer, but her organization continued on (72).

Mrs. Hoffman's emphasis upon "Freedom of Choice" in
cancer treatment echoed the constantly reiterated dominant
theme of another organization which had been established
eight years before she founded the IACVF. The National
Health Federation was founded in 1955 (73, 74). Moving
spirit in its creation was Fred J. Hart, a California promoter of health devices who had just been enjoined by Food
and Drug Administration initiative from distributing them
in interstate commerce. Other NHF founding fathers also had
encountered legal restraints, some spending time in jail,
for false claims about devices, dietary wares, and so-called
cancer treatments. One of Harry Hoxsey's lawyers became the

Federation's first legal representative in Washington. The
Federation developed into a powerful league linking the various segments of health unorthodoxy. They held up each
other's spirits and sought new converts at frequent meetings,
developed skillful propaganda playing on public anxieties
and frustrations, grew adept at pressure politics, mobiliz-
ing the faithful for letter-writing campaigns and confronta-
tion lobbying. Hart and Krebs both testified against the
California cancer law, and the Federation welcomed Laetrile
supporters to its ranks and gave their cause strong support.
Condemning overweening and bumbling bureaucracy for administering health laws to favor the medical establishment, the
NHF pleaded for patient freedom of choice so that each ail-
ing person might treat himself from amongst unorthodoxy's
abundant catalog of wares. The Federation journal pictured
Washington and Lincoln on its cover over the caption, "They
Too Fought for Liberty Against Great Odds." These criticisms
of governmental actions in the health field mounted amidst
the growing broader disillusion with governmental policy
resulting from the war in Vietnam.

The distorted Laetrile version of the FDA's rejection
of McNaughton's IND received widespread coverage in the publications of unorthodoxy and in the sensationalist press
(75). A barrage of angry mail bombarded Washington. FDA's
police state tactics, charged one protester, "reduce[d]
Hitler and Stalin to the status of small time hoodlums" (76).

Mail deluged the Congress as well as the FDA (77). The
National Health Federation Bulletin had explicitly urged this
action (78). Representative Lawrence H. Fountain, after
committee hearings, brought pressure on Elliot Richardson,
Secretary of Health, Education, and Welfare, to sponsor further evaluation of Laetrile's efficacy (79). The FDA checked
its own internal judgment by soliciting external expert
opinion. A panel of independent cancer specialists was
assembled, which reviewed the data submitted in McNaughton's
application, heard face-to-face what McNaughton and Burk had
to say, sought whatever new information Laetrile physicians
like Contreras might have to offer, then concluded that the
sum total of evidence did not warrant testing Laetrile on
humans. Further rodent tests in recognized independent laboratories, the committee held, might be desirable. The
Secretary considered the conclusions of FDA's ad hoc committee valid (63, 80). National Cancer Institute tests on mice
had offered no promise of Laetrile's effectiveness, and no
new NCI tests seemed worth undertaking. That Institute, however, the Secretary said, would recognize grant applications
for further testing from qualified independent investigators.

Secretary Richardson reported his judgments to Congressman
Fountain who did not continue to press the issue. A bill
introduced into the House by another member, to authorize
research on and testing of non-toxic substances for the diagnosis, treatment, and prevention of cancer, made no headway
(81).

     Regulatory pressure on Laetrile promoters did not sub-
side. In 1971 the state of California began a criminal case
against Ernst Krebs, Jr., charging him with practicing medicine without a license and, aided by his brother Byron, an
osteopathic physician, with distributing a prohibited drug
(82, 83, 84). Two years later the brothers pleaded nolo con-
tendere to violating the state cancer act's taboo on Laetrile.
The judge fined them and placed them on probation. The terms
required them to obey all city, state, and federal laws, especially the cancer treatment provisions of the California
code, and forbade Krebs, Jr., to practice medicine without a
license. California took further legal steps as well. A case
against Mary Whelchel sought to impede the turning wheels of
an accelerating "underground railroad" which assembled cancer
victims from all over the nation in a boarding house on the
United States side of the border, then ran them across to
Tijuana for Laetrile treatment in Dr. Contreras' flourishing
operation (84, 85). In 1971, Mrs. Whelchel was convicted of
delivering an illegal compound for treating cancer, fined,
and, as a term of her probation, was forbidden to transport
anyone to Mexico. (It should be noted, however, that this
conviction was set aside two years later.)

The Appeal to Freedom

     Such relentless regulation coupled with scant success
from the epistolary campaign in Washington sped changes already launched that remade Laetrile's self-image, the explanation for its therapeutic action, indications for its use,
the strategy and tactics of its promotion, even its very
name. Andrew McNaughton remained commanding general, but
became an officer in exile. In 1974 his reputation in his
Canadian homeland suffered a blow when a judge convicted him
of conspiring fraudulently to affect the market price of a
mining stock (86). The United States, with Laetrile under
attack on both state and federal levels, must have seemed increasingly hostile. McNaughton took up residence in Tijuana.
The press credited his foundation with sponsoring both manufacturing and clinical facilities for Laetrile in the Mexican
city (36), stations at the underground railroad's terminus.
The railroad began to run the other way, carrying smuggled
Mexican Laetrile into the U.S.A. (87).

McNaughton thus continued, as a reporter put it, "more than any other man . . . the driving force behind the Laetrile movement" (88). In this third period, however, McNaughton in exile gained powerful allies of great leadership potential in the United States. This chain of events began in 1972 when a California general practitioner, Dr. John A. Richardson, was arrested at his Albany clinic, charged with prescribing Laetrile in violation of the state's anti-quackery law (89). The dramatic arrest, filmed on television cameras, involved policemen with drawn guns and a thorough search of the premises. The physician spent a brief time in jail. A trial before a judge, finding Richardson guilty, was quashed on appeal. Two jury trials followed, both ending with jurors split (36, 90). Eventually the California Board of Medical Quality Assurance revoked Dr. Richardson's license to practice medicine on grounds of "Gross negligence and incompetence" (91, 92).

Richardson's initial arrest upset some of his fellow members of the John Birch Society. Such dedicated disciples of freedom-from-government doctrine saw in Richardson's plight a prime example of bureaucratic oppression. Led by Robert W. Bradford of Los Altos, a small group of ultraconservatives founded yet another organization to help Laetrile's besieged prescribers (93). Bradford was a nuclear technician on the Stanford University staff, working on the building of a linear accelerator for research in subatomic physics. Poised, articulate, skilled at organization, Bradford, aided by equally dedicated associates, quickly made a success of the new Committee for Freedom of Choice in Cancer Therapy (36, 94, 95). In 1975 he gave up his Stanford job to devote full time to the Committee and to Laetrile. Ties with the nation's already existing conservative network surely helped immensely in the speed with which the Committee established local branches. By 1977 Bradford claimed five hundred chapters with some 35,000 members.

The Committee and its allies focused upon freedom, making any governmental interference with a cancer sufferer's right to take any remedy available seem a violation of the Constitution and the fundamental rights of man. Thus an atmosphere of high principle infused the zealous campaigning in Laetrile's behalf. Laetrile's opponents, in the Committee's propaganda, constituted a selfish conspiracy of those involved in orthodox cancer research and therapy, futilely cutting, burning, and poisoning their victims, and rejecting hopeful treatments like Laetrile for fear of doing themselves out of their jobs. The Committee showed great ingenuity at making their message widely known. They employed meetings,

films, pamphlets, paperback books, quickly triggered letter-
writing campaigns, and the assembling of the faithful for
legislative hearings. Full-time crusaders sought out cancer
victims and urged Laetrile upon them and upon members of their
families (96). Counsel could be given as to how to get to
Contreras' clinic in Mexico or how to acquire Laetrile in the
United States. Indeed, some Committee leaders, including
President Bradford himself, allegedly at great personal profit,
engaged in a conspiracy to smuggle Laetrile in from Mexico and,
with much surreptitious ingenuity, distribute it within the
United States. After a three-month trial in 1977, Bradford,
Dr. Richardson, and others were convicted of this conspiracy;
the Court of Appeals for the Ninth Circuit confirmed the con-
victions (97). McNaughton, also indicted, pleaded guilty (87).

Laetrile in the 1970s assumed a different character from
the chemotherapeutic Laetrile with which the Krebs began. In
1963, in a letter to the Food and Drug Administration, Dr.
Krebs had asserted: "The cyanogenetic glucosides belong to
the nutritional vitamins and should not be classified as
drugs" (98). Here appears the earliest reference encountered
in the file to Laetrile's future destiny. Already, Krebs,
Jr., had committed himself, as part of his probation, not to
distribute Laetrile as a drug. Perhaps both father and son
had begun to wonder if legal restrictions might not be less
stringent under the food sections of the law. Such a shift
in Laetrile's status would require a modification of the prevailing chemotherapeutic explanations of Laetrile's mode of
action. Shortly Krebs, Jr., published a pamphlet, not really
retreating, but adding the suggestion that Laetrile could be
characterized as a pro-vitamin for B-12. The pamphlet bore
the title, "Cancer Is a Deficiency Disease" (21).

As regulatory actions mounted, Krebs, Jr., in 1970
brought his pamphlet title to full flower. In an article in
the Journal of Applied Nutrition he asserted that Laetrile
and other "nitrolosides" made up a true vitamin which he denominated B-17 (99). Vitamin B-17, he wrote, amounted to a
cancer-protective factor. Moreover, Krebs asserted, in this
"new vitamin . . . all of us are severely deficient." Cancer
could be cured by massive injections of the vitamin. Cancer
could also be prevented by smaller quantities, made from de-
fatted apricot kernels, regularly taken by mouth. Four years
before the appearance of this article Dr. Krebs had begun to
distribute an oral dosage form of Laetrile (100). Now that
form became popular, widely publicized by McNaughton, as co-
therapy with injections of Laetrile in cancer treatment and,
among perfectly healthy people, as a presumed preventive.
Chewing unprocessed apricot kernels bought at health food
stores also came into vogue.

If one were interested in Laetrile as a commercial venture, one might anticipate several advantages from this combination of new directions. Vitamin status for a product, one could argue and hope, might bring some immunity from actions under the drug provisions of both state and federal law. Moreover, the concept of cancer prevention would certainly elicit broad public interest, for of all threats, including war, Americans feared cancer most. Potential sales of a preventive could be enormous. And, if to the popular mind the word "cancer" bore ominous overtones, the word "vitamin" evoked glamorous reverberations of buoyant health (101). Americans had mounted to a new plateau of concern about their health, accompanied by a wide variety of approaches toward do-it-yourself safeguarding, by no means all of them sound. Health food marketers, including National Health Federation members, both agitated the public's concern about health and oversold the need for vitamin supplementation (102).

Nutritional scientists repeatedly denied that Laetrile fulfilled any of the criteria for a true vitamin (103, 104, 105). "In short," summed up a veteran vitamin researcher, Dr. Thomas H. Jukes, "nothing could be less like a vitamin than laetrile" (106). Despite such criticism, Laetrile's vendors continued to assert this claim. In testifying in 1977 before Senator Edward Kennedy's Subcommittee on Health, Ernst Krebs, Jr., termed Laetrile "a scientific revolution as profound as the germ theory of disease . . . and the Copernican theory" (107). What Vitamin C is to scurvy, niacin to pellagra, and Vitamin D to rickets, he suggested, Vitamin B-17 is to cancer. If every American took Laetrile regularly, Dr. Richardson told the subcommittee, "in 20 years cancer would be relegated to the dusty pages of history."

To make amygdalin accessible for regular self-dosage by the American public, Laetrile's sponsors displayed much marketing skill. In 1972 there appeared in California a consumer product bearing the trade name Seventeen. Just in front of the name on the carton came a picture of a bee. A McNaughton Foundation representative offered a reporter from a San Jose newspaper a chance to interview the noted cancer specialist, Dean Burk, who happened to be visiting the Bay area (108, 109). By this route Burk's praise for the new food supplement found its way into the press. Bee-Seventeen, Burk said, contained three percent Laetrile, thirty percent protein, fifty percent unsaturated fats, with the remainder minerals. The powder was to be taken daily with juices or milk. Laetrile, Burk told the reporter, could both prevent and cure cancer, but no medical claims were being made in

behalf of Bee-Seventeen. It was offered for sale solely as
a food.

Such a ruse did not protect the product from action by
the Food and Drug Administration. The manufacturers of Bee-
Seventeen were enjoined from distributing what the court
termed both an unapproved food additive and a misbranded
drug (110). Other amygdalin-containing products, like
Aprikern, though devoid of therapeutic claims in their labeling, were also barred from the marketplace (111).

Laetrile's champions not only propagated their vitamin
gospel with aggressive vigor; they also took the offensive
against their critics in other ways. Oppressed by federal
food and drug law and by the California anti-quackery statute, the Laetrile coalition turned its attention to legislative chambers. Several efforts to repeal the efficacy provision in the California law failed (112). In the national
Congress, Laetrile supporters favored a bill introduced by
Representative Steven D. Symms of Idaho which would have
repealed the provision of the Kefauver-Harris Act requiring
that new drugs be proved effective before being permitted on
the market (113, 114). This bill gained some 140 co-sponsors
in the House but made no progress toward enactment.

Laetrile's major legislative push aimed at persuading
state legislatures to pass laws legalizing the extract made
from apricot kernels. Bills differed in substance from
state to state, although most would at least permit physicians to prescribe Laetrile for patients certified as terminally ill of cancer (115). Cancer specialists pointed to
the great difficulty in achieving any satisfactory definition
of the word "terminal" (116). Alaska enacted the first such
law in September 1976, and within two years sixteen other
states had followed suit. Other legislatures pondered Laetrile bills and defeated them. The deliberative bodies in
Indiana, Illinois, and Rhode Island enacted their measures
over vetoes by the governors (117, 118). In New York, two
years in succession the governor's veto held.

The scenarios in the several states had much in common
(119). A cooperative assemblyman introduced a bill at the
request of a constituent. In due course the health committee held hearings. The hearings, replete with drama, became
newsworthy happenings, recorded by television cameras, widely
reported in the press. In some states, orthodoxy and unorthodoxy got equal time in number of testifying witnesses.
In other states, pro-Laetrile sentiment was dominant. In
news coverage, unorthodoxy--the underdog, the challenger--

received the greater play. Members of The Committee for
Freedom of Choice in Cancer Therapy turned out in force.
Wearing campaign buttons, they packed the galleries, intense,
completely absorbed. Depending on the strictness of the
rules imposed, Laetrile's friends either shouted or murmured
praise for pro-Laetrile testimony, and heaped imprecations,
either loudly or sotto voce, upon spokesmen from the state
medical society, nearby universities, the American Cancer
Society, the Food and Drug Administration, who explicated
Laetrile's unproven status. The Laetrile lobby produced living testimonials claiming to demonstrate the contrary. After
my operation--so the pattern went--my doctors gave me only a
year to live, but I took Laetrile and here I am three years
later, speaking before you legislators. The main thrust,
however, of Laetrile spokesmen, often the national leaders of
the movement, fell upon freedom of choice. State legislators
had their own problems with the powerful federal presence,
and might listen with sympathy to constituents blasting segments of the Washington bureaucracy. In any case, pleaded
Laetrile witnesses in many states, only a little freedom was
being sought, freedom for the dying, under a doctor's direction, to try Laetrile as a last resort.

After the hearings came continued pressure upon legislators, through conversations and a massive deluge of mail.
Occasionally, if the terms of initial bills seemed too broad
for acceptance, successive versions would follow with ever
weaker provisions, until skeptical assemblymen would consider the measure too innocuous to matter and could thus
satisfy both their consciences and the demands of those who
had sent in the preponderance of mail.

No matter how weak the laws enacted, each one, announced to the nation through growing media coverage, contributed
to bandwagon psychology, giving the imprimatur of another
state's approval to Laetrile. To the ordinary citizen, sanction might equate with efficacy. Thus each new law enhancing
Laetrile's prestige made it seem like legitimate therapy to
victims of cancer and their families, including those victims
whose cancer had just been diagnosed. And each law, making
a specific exemption of Laetrile, dealt a new blow to the
theory behind the federal law, which many states had imi-
tated, that promoters of new drugs must prove them efficacious and safe before they could be marketed. The Kefauver
law, moreover, demanded a high standard for proving efficacy,
the results of adequate and well-controlled studies, not random cases proclaiming benefit, whether presented in paperback
book or in testimony at committee hearing.

The state laws, however, did not negate the national law, and Laetrile remained illegal in interstate commerce. It was reported that McNaughton, allied with Bradford in a new John Beard Research Institute in Palo Alto, hoped to set up plants to manufacture Laetrile and clinics to dispense it within states enacting favorable laws (120), although these projects did not move rapidly forward. And in Illinois at least, where legal use of Laetrile was hedged in with many restrictions, the pattern set by the law has not been much employed (121). Rather, black market Laetrile has continued to be vended in the most dangerously careless way. A Chicago reporter told of buying Laetrile surreptitiously from a foot doctor downstate who asked no medical questions (122).

A second legal route for Laetrile prescribing, this one breaching the ban on interstate commerce, developed from action in the federal courts. As the Laetrile forces undertook a counter-offensive against regulation on the legislative front, so also did they on the judicial front. The key case in the campaign centered on Glen L. Rutherford, a manufacturer's representative who lived in Conway Springs, Kansas (123). Upon receiving a medical diagnosis that he suffered from a cancerous polyp, Rutherford refused radical surgery of the larger bowel. Instead he went to Dr. Contreras' clinic in Tijuana. The physician in charge of Rutherford's case later wrote a federal judge that Rutherford was treated with Laetrile and proteolytic enzymes, and then the remaining polyp was "cauterized" (123). Cancer specialists indicate that the excision of a polyp of this type solves the problem in a high proportion of cancer cases (124).

Upon returning home, Rutherford sought to ensure himself of a continuing supply of Laetrile. He joined a law suit already begun, became the sole surviving plaintiff, and in 1975 won from the United States District Court in Oklahoma an injunction against federal regulators which permitted him and other terminally ill cancer patients to import from Mexico a limited amount of the drug for their personal use (123). Judge Luther Bohanon insisted that each patient present a physician's affidavit certifying to the stage of illness and specifying the quantity of Laetrile needed to be imported.

Upon appeal of the Rutherford case, the United States Court of Appeals for the Tenth Circuit upheld the injunction (125). The court also instructed Judge Bohanon to require the Food and Drug Administration to develop an administrative record on two points contested in the case: whether or not Laetrile was a "new drug" as defined by law, and whether or not it was exempt from premarketing approval requirements by

reason of being "grandfathered." FDA complied. In its proceeding, the agency received four hundred written statements
from friends and foes of Laetrile and held in May 1977 two
days of public hearings in Kansas City (126). Jammed with
Laetrile supporters, these hearings had the emotional flavor
of hearings in the states (105). Cheers greeted pro-Laetrile
speakers, boos and hisses their opponents. To one distinguished scientist present, "the affair appeared to be a con-
frontation between two cultures. One side was characterized
by the voice of science--skeptical, analytical, orderly, but
sometimes bluntly critical and uncompromising. The other
side faced the situation with fervor, passion, conviction,
revolt against logic, all emotionally expressed. They
seemed to willfully reject distasteful facts" (105).

Food and Drug Commissioner Donald Kennedy and his staff
turned their court-appointed responsibility into a comprehensive review of Laetrile, as thorough, broad-gauged, and
insightful an analysis of a highly promoted but unorthodox
drug as could be found in the American literature (21). Besides answering the court-posed issues--Laetrile had not
been "grandfathered" under either the 1938 or 1962 law; experts did not consider it either safe or effective for its
prescribed uses--the report discussed other significant matters relating to Laetrile. Laetrile's composition and identity would be difficult to define, the report stated, because
so many different chemical entities had appeared under that
name in both the literature printed about and the products
distributed as Laetrile. The Commissioner countered the
various claims made for Laetrile's effectiveness in cancer,
disputing the shifting theories, remarking the inadequate
anecdotal character of pro-Laetrile case reporting, and citing the lack of promise in numerous well controlled animal
studies that had been made by the National Cancer Institute
and private cancer research centers. The few animal tests
interpreted as favorable to Laetrile by Dean Burk and others,
the report criticized directly, concluding that Laetrile had
failed "to show any effect in the animal system." The document found the nature of Laetrile's appeal in the psychology
of patients and their loved ones caught in the crushing cancer crisis. The "disparagement of conventional therapy," the
Commissioner stated, "a bulwark of the campaigns of Laetrile
proponents, is perhaps the most morally reprehensible aspect
of the pattern of the drug's promotion." This disparagement
led sufferers away from proven remedies, that might offer
some chance, to almost certain disaster. Even short delays
could mean the difference between life and death.

Commissioner Kennedy met the "freedom of choice" argument head on. Congress had decided, he noted, "that the

absolute freedom to choose an ineffective drug was properly
surrendered in exchange for the freedom from the danger to
each person's health and well-being from the sale and use of
worthless drugs." In any case, the choice to use Laetrile,
made in an atmosphere of double stress, compounded from fear
of disease and from the zeal of Laetrile advocates, with
seldom any "rational laying out of competing arguments," can
seldom be properly described as free.

The Commissioner's conclusions and all their buttressing
evidence did not persuade the Oklahoma judge. He ruled that
Laetrile was exempt from the need for pre-market approval and
forbade the Food and Drug Administration from interfering
with its importation and transport in interstate commerce or
with its use by licensed medical practitioners in treating
cancer patients (127). Again the FDA appealed.

When the Tenth Circuit considered FDA's appeal of this
new Rutherford decision, the judges cut back markedly on the
District Court's liberality toward Laetrile, but still
authorized its use for a restricted segment of the population
(128). Ruling in July 1978, the appellate judges concluded
that the law's taboo against unsafe and ineffective drugs
did not apply to people who were dying. Therefore, patients
whose physicians would certify that they were terminally ill
with cancer could legally import Laetrile--but only for intravenous injections, not in its oral form.

This last proviso revealed that the Court of Appeals
was taking into account, as the District Court had not,
evidence of amygdalin's toxicity when taken by mouth. Evidence submitted to the Commissioner's review, testimony
given before Senator Kennedy's subcommittee, and stories in
the press cited severe poisonings and even deaths from the
ingestion of Laetrile tablets and apricot kernels (21, 129,
130, 131, 132). Enzymes in the gastrointestinal tract split
the amygdalin molecule and released its cyanide.

The Tenth Circuit did not heed other evidence submitted
to it with the FDA's appeal, that the long-vaunted claims
made in behalf of injectable Laetrile's non-toxicity might
not be completely true. Little research had been undertaken
on Laetrile's action when injected into the body. Some
physicians began to report unfortunate consequences, sur-
mising that many such adverse effects had earlier occurred
but had been blamed not upon the treatment but upon the
disease (133).

That the dying should be barred from the law's protective mantle, Commissioner Kennedy deemed a "remarkable find-

ing" indeed, and he urged an appeal of the Tenth Circuit's
opinion to the Supreme Court (134). In August 1978 the
Commissioner thought his hand strengthened when the Court
of Appeals for the Seventh Circuit rendered an anti-Laetrile
decision. In 1977 FDA had seized apricot kernels, partially
processed kernels, and empty capsules intended for filling
with Laetrile at perhaps the largest processing plant in
the United States, a former dairy in Manitowoc, Wisconsin.
Later the company, which had sold two million dollars worth
of its illegal product, was enjoined from continuing its
business (135). On appeal, the Seventh Circuit ruled that
Laetrile could properly be excluded from interstate commerce
until it should be proven safe and effective (136). In due
course the Supreme Court could be expected to decide between
the contrary opinions of the Tenth and Seventh Circuits (137).

Other con and pro decisions marked Laetrile's increasingly litigious history. In California, the state's effort
to restrain Laetrile practitioners ran into a snag. A state
appeals court called the California cancer law unconstitutional, ruling that the state had no power to deny doctors
the right to use non-toxic unorthodox cancer treatments
(138). The state Supreme Court in 1978 granted a petition for
review of this decision (139). In Georgia, a jury exonerated
one of the most notable personages in the ranks of Laetrile
proponents. Larry P. McDonald, physician and member of the
John Birch Society and of the United States Congress, had
prescribed only Laetrile for a patient's cancer (140). When
the man died, his family sued for malpractice. The jury
decided not so, yet feeling sympathy for the widow decided
that she should be reimbursed for the expense of her dead
husband's treatment.

The Food and Drug Administration continued seizing im-
ports of Laetrile from Mexico and from Germany not protected
by court-ordered physician affidavits swearing that the drug
was intended for a particular patient who was terminally ill.
Moreover, some samples offered for import turned out to be
not amygdalin at all, but a dangerous fever reducer; other
samples were contaminated with fungus (141, 142). Indeed,
even the affidavit system itself, the FDA soon charged, had
become a cloak for fraud (143). Reporters visiting Tijuana
observed stacks of presigned affidavits available for the asking to Laetrile purchasers (122). Hitherto Laetrile smuggling, as revealed in the trial at which Dr. Richardson and
Bradford had been convicted, had been an underground operation. Now, the government alleged in a seizure action, the
druggist at a Baltimore pharmacy had manipulated the affidavit system for his own profit (144, 145). He had obtained

affidavits from a physician and had filled them in for the maximum importable amount of Laetrile, using the names of cancer patients who had in fact ordered smaller quantities or none at all. The druggist had then sold the surplus to other patients, sometimes getting the authorized release and sometimes not. A judge upheld the validity of the seizure, but, pending a Supreme Court decision, would not order the seized Laetrile destroyed.

The extensive litigation and the legislative battles in the states made Laetrile an issue of national interest and debate. News magazines carried cover stories (37). Television--including the program "60 Minutes" (146)--looked at Laetrile. The press kept tabulated track of contests in the states. Conservative columnists, most notably James J. Kilpatrick, attracted to the freedom of choice theme, repeatedly gave Laetrile users a prestigious boost (147). The promoters intensified their own publicity. Paperback successors followed Kittler's original success: G. Edward Griffin's World Without Cancer in 1974 (148); Mike Culbert's Freedom from Cancer in 1976 (149); John Richardson's Laetrile Case Histories (90) and Robert Bradford's Now That You Have Cancer in 1977 (150). A majority of American citizens, according to a Louis Harris poll, thought decriminalization of Laetrile would be a good idea (151). Some Laetrile leaders sounded smug at their success.

"Rest assured, gentlemen," Bradford told Senator Kennedy's subcommittee, "that the people demand Laetrile. . . And they are going to get it whether Big Brother wants it or not. . . . [W]e cannot expect that thousands of American cancer sufferers are going to wait for more long years, while the Federal Government fiddle-faddles through animal tests and more redtape. . . Do we really want another American civil war?" (152).

So disturbed became the state of the mass mind that a segment of sober opinion, unbelievers in Laetrile's efficacy, concluded that the speediest way to quiet public clamor would be to let Laetrile's worthlessness be proved either by widespread use or in a series of well controlled clinical trials in humans conducted by investigators of unimpeachable integrity and skill. Some scientists, indeed, believe that any drug should be tested for which suggestive evidence exists, even hearsay, that the drug might be of benefit. To test Laetrile in humans would breach the prevailing system, which puts the burden of proof upon a new drug's sponsor. Such a step, further, would fly in the face of the weight of animal evidence. The major pro-Laetrile

animal experiments, announced in 1977 at a National Health
Federation meeting by Harold W. Manner, a zoologist at Loyola University in Chicago (153, 154), have received severe
criticism on the grounds of inadequate methodology (155).
Human trials with Laetrile, therefore, posed grave ethical
questions respecting patient rights and the value of expend-
ing limited resources available for testing in such a way
(156). But so dangerous seemed the consequences of the
spirit behind the new Laetrile state laws that some commen-
tators, both laymen and physicians, resorted to the forbidden
fruit argument. The way to dampen "Laetrilomania," suggested
F. J. Ingelfinger, distinguished editor of the New England
Journal of Medicine, might be to reduce the glamor derived
from its illicit status by making it freely available, and
then keeping accurate records of patient experience (157).
The editors of the New York Times took a similar tolerant
approach toward Laetrile distribution (158). Charles G.
Moertel of the Mayo Clinic favored a less extreme course:
if Laetrile's sponsors would not assume their legal obliga-
tions, then reputable scientists must undertake the task.
"The only established means of proving a drug effective or
ineffective, safe or unsafe[,] is by a properly designed,
tightly controlled clinical trial" (159).

Officials at the National Cancer Institute reluctantly
reached the same conclusion. If such action had to come,
FDA Commissioner Kennedy argued at Senator Kennedy's hearing,
at least all parties must agree on the specific chemical formula, among the many that had been posited and marketed, of
the "Laetrile" to be tested (160). Senator Kennedy labored
diligently throughout the hearing and believed he had achieved
a consensus on this point which included Laetrile's promoters.
Tests would weigh the merit of amygdalin (161).

After careful review of the situation, National Cancer
Institute officials decided not to launch human trials
immediately, but to undertake a retrospective study of
patients who, according to their physicians, might have bene-
fited objectively from the use of Laetrile (162). From the
purportedly 70,000 patients in the United States who had been
treated with Laetrile, the NCI hoped to get full enough
records to permit analysis of two or three hundred cases. In
quest of such records a much publicized appeal went forth to
the more than 400,000 physicians and other health professionals in the nation. The director of the project sought
to persuade the Laetrile inner ring of leadership to urge
physicians active in Laetrile prescribing to submit case
records (163).

In the end, however, only ninety-three cancer cases were

submitted for evaluation, only twenty-two of them concerning
patients who had been treated with Laetrile alone for whom
the records were adequate for appraisal (164). A panel of
twelve cancer experts stated that under Laetrile treatment
apparently seven of the patients had worsened, nine had remained the same, and six had responded favorably, two with
complete and four with partial remissions. These conclusions, the reviewers granted, had to be taken with a grain
of salt because of the possible "submission of incorrect
clinical interpretations, falsified data and intentional
or unintentional omission of data." Nor had the review been
designed to discover patients who had not responded to Laetrile. Nonetheless, more than two hundred physicians had
volunteered evidence about more than a thousand patients who
had shown no beneficial response.

After further review, the National Cancer Institute re-
vived its earlier decision to undertake a clinical trial of
amygdalin in some 150 to three hundred terminal cancer patients. Dr. Arthur Upton, NCI director, announced the plan
in September 1978, expressing hope that the outcome would
resolve the debate over Laetrile "once and for all" (165).

Such optimism seemed scarcely warranted. Laetrile proponents, while publicly appealing for testing, had been
customarily reluctant or unable to provide complete data on
patients for evaluation. The FDA's request for clinical
records to Dr. Contreras and to a German experimenter, Dr.
Hans Nieper, had not brought in usable material. Nieper
submitted no data at all, and Contreras' case records, when
evaluated by NCI scientists, showed no patient benefits as-
cribable to Laetrile (166). Contreras, in fact, insisted to
a reporter that employing his clinic for purposes of research
would be unethical (167). Nor had a whole succession of
animal experiments, which to established cancer researchers
offered no hint of Laetrile's efficacy, satisfied Laetrile's
proponents, who sought to reinterpret a few such trials in
a way favorable to their product (168).

From the beginning, indeed, as a basic premise, Laetrile's supporters questioned the validity of experiments
conducted by experimenters who did not share faith in the
theories supporting Laetrile's value. Pro-Laetrile physicians must direct the clinical trials, Krebs, Jr., had
told the California Cancer Commission in 1952, or he would
not provide Laetrile for experimentation (23). In 1977
Krebs made essentially the same point: those inside and
outside the Laetrile movement "do not necessarily speak the
same language" (107). Each dwells "in a different universe"
(60). Unless, a pro-Laetrile physician told the Kennedy

subcommittee, the NCI study should be conducted "in the way
that the proponents of Laetrile . . . are urging that it be
done," then "it will be an absolute sham" (107). Robert
Bradford echoed these sentiments: "the protocols that exist
for orthodox therapy are not applicable[,] for the most part,
to metabolic therapy and Laetrile" (95). Traditional oncologists, for example, held that the removal or reduction
in the size of a neoplasm measured the success of therapy,
whereas espousers of Vitamin B-17, believing cancer to be a
deficiency disease, considered the size of the lump irrele-
vant. "You do not and cannot expect to get results from
laetrile treatment," Bradford said at the Kansas City hearing, "unless you are a trained metabolic physician" (169).

Commissioner Donald Kennedy wondered if some maneuvers
by Laetrile's promoters might not be intended for the purpose of disparaging test results adverse to the drug (160).
"[I]n sifting the strange mixture of nomenclature, alleged
chemical identity, and proposed mechanism of action that
comprises Laetrile's record of the past twenty-five years,"
Dr. Kennedy said, "one becomes gradually convinced that
these uncertainties are not accidental. They provide an
effective cover for the promoters, since failure to achieve
a result can always be attributed to having used the wrong
material and arguments against one hypothesis of action can
always be met by embracing another."

During the Vitamin B-17 period, the increasing stress
upon "total metabolic therapy" marked another change in
approach to the promotion of Laetrile. In treating cancer,
according to the new doctrine, Laetrile alone could not be
relied upon. While Vitamin B-17 held the indispensable
place, it needed to be administered as part of a complex
program involving a multitude of variables (150). The
other parts consisted of diet, exercise, rest, detoxifica-
tion, minerals, enzymes, vitamins A, C, and E, and that
other major Krebs' promotion, Vitamin B-15 or pangamic acid.
A patient might require "several dozen tablets every day."

In Bradford's book, Now That You Have Cancer, he likened the metabolic program to a crown containing nine jewels,
with Laetrile "the crown jewel within that diadem" (150).
Such a "total approach," combining an attack on the cancer,
a bolstering of the body, and a positive mental attitude,
metabolic physicians held, provided "the best chance to
control cancer." If the metabolic doctrine bolstered Laetrile with a host of attendant therapies, the system also
expanded Laetrile's prowess beyond cancer. In a book entitled How You Can Beat the Killer Diseases, Harold W.
Harper accorded Laetrile a role in preventing and treating

a broad range of other ailments, including diabetes, emphysema, arthritis, and cardiovascular disease (170).

The diversified regimen of metabolic therapy certainly complicated the problem of evaluating in human trials Laetrile's role as a possible therapeutic agent for cancer, and made second-guessing of results inevitable. Nonetheless, the National Cancer Institute's Dr. Upton stated that, in devising the Institute's experiments, he would "not rule out the possibility of looking at combinations" of Laetrile and high-potency vitamins (165). Laetrile's advocates greeted the NCI's retrospective review as "Laetrile's biggest breakthrough," because "from now on the myth as to the 'officially' observed lack of validity in Laetrile has been destroyed" (171). Yet Bradford had told the Kansas City hearing that no "effective agreed upon protocol" for a study of cancer under metabolic therapy could be set up (169). Whatever a NCI trial might show, disputations between advocates of orthodoxy and champions of unorthodoxy seemed certain to continue.

The Pattern of Cancer Unorthodoxies

Health quackery has flourished since that ancient day when, as Voltaire put it, the first knave met the first fool. Through most of American history, nourished by the Enlightenment concepts of the Revolutionary generation, the presence of quackery has been acknowledged but its status has been considered transitory. When medical science had expanded its horizons a little further, when the populace had received a little more schooling, when the Congress had enacted another protective law, then would quackery vanish, consigned to the museum of outmoded delusions. Certainly through the Progressive period at the beginning of our own century, such optimism sustained itself (172). When the Pure Food and Drugs Act became law in 1906, the New York Times editorialized: "the purity and honesty of the . . . medicines of the people are guaranteed" (173).

As the twentieth century has proceeded, despite enhanced medical science, more universal schooling, and a great increase in social legislation, observers have grown less confident about predicting quackery's imminent demise. The course of events and the pathways of philosophy both have chilled such naive optimism. The doctrine of inevitable progress fell under the impact of a series of terrible wars. Faith in the inherent goodness of human nature, battered by new philosophical perspectives, crumbled under the revelations from the Nazi concentration camps. Belief in education as a panacea withered. Science-technology

inventiveness did continue to produce wondrous products for
mankind's benefit but also devised nuclear weapons and
polluted the environment. Modern industrial civilization
struck many people as part of the cause for burgeoning un-
happiness, Ernst Krebs, Jr., among them. At the Kansas City
hearing, Krebs expressed abhorrence for "the horrible on-
slaught of technology blindly impinging upon the fragile
flesh that contains our flame of life" (60). Some disturbed
souls sought to return to nature. Pressing upon this long
developing crisis of confidence came Vietnam, an unpopular
and unsuccessful war that put generations at each other's
throats, and Watergate, seeming proof of what some voices
had long been crying, that blame for the discontents of
civilization could be laid upon leadership.

Such an atmosphere induces irrational approaches to
fundamental problems. The disillusioned, questing for new
faith, are terribly vulnerable to false prophets. Distrust
of established authorities encompasses all those who have
traditionally sought to protect the public from charlatanry.
The medical profession suffers suspicion, including the
specialists within it concerned with cancer. In a behavioral
survey sponsored by the Food and Drug Administration and
other federal agencies, it was revealed that forty-two percent of American adults would not be persuaded by almost
unanimous expert opinion that an unorthodox "cancer cure"
held out false hope (101).

Cancer quackery in America goes back to the earliest
days. In colonial times one purported cure consisted of
alleged "Chinese Stones" vended by a self-styled Frenchman
who hawked his wares from town to town (174). At the beginning of this century, the first major case lost by the
government under the 1906 law had aimed at suppressing Dr.
Johnson's Mild Combination Treatment for Cancer (175). By
mid-century unorthodox cancer promotions loomed largest
among the illegal operations which regulatory agencies
sought to control.

Basic to this circumstance were both the impact and the
image of cancer in our society. With the decline of infec-
tious diseases as a cause of death, due to sanitation,
vaccines, and chemotherapy, cancer had risen to second place
in the mortality lists. The 1900 death rate for malignant
neoplasms was 64 per 100,000 deaths, the 1977 estimated rate
177 (176). On the disease and death front, cancer had moved
to the center of public attention. A sense of urgency led
to an all-out attack, with billions of dollars appropriated
by the Congress in imitation of the nation's venture into

outer space, in an effort to conquer cancer once and for all. But the enemy proved to be too complex for such a battle plan. Despite many advances, failure to fulfill the central promise brought new disillusionment (177).

Yet the image of cancer may be an even more important force for quackery than its factual circumstances. Heart deaths exceed cancer deaths, but no wave of cardiovascular cures has surfaced similar to those in the cancer field. That centuries ago cancer began to acquire a hostile and terrifying image may be deduced from the word "cancer" itself, derived from the Greek work for crab. The crawling spread of cancer, gradual but mainly relentless, whether external and observable or internal and secretive, through the centuries appeared to be, and indeed generally did amount to, a sentence of death. This image hangs on, a powerful force in men's minds, a force not adequately revised by the victories orthodoxy increasingly has won. In our mythology, Susan Sontag has written, cancer has become a "cosmic disease: the emblem of all the destructive, alien powers to which the organism is host . . . [C]ancer is thought of as a disease of the contamination of the whole world" (178). "As long as a particular disease is treated as an evil, invincible predator, not just a disease," she states, "most people with cancer will indeed be demoralized by learning what disease they have." And Sontag cites Karl Menninger to the effect that "the very word 'cancer' is said to kill some patients." This deeply imbedded fear is constantly revivified in the lurid tracts and the camp meeting oratory of orthodoxy's opponents.

Four major unorthodoxies have emerged in the United States during the last half century. First, a Detroit physician, William F. Koch, proclaimed his newly discovered Glyoxilide an anti-toxin for cancer. Each ampul, costing $25, Koch said, contained one part Glyoxilide to one trillion parts of water. Three thousand American health practitioners bought and administered the purported chemical, charging up to $300 per injection (179).

Second, a former coal miner, Harry Hoxsey, after treating external cancers with caustics here and there in Illinois, made his way to Dallas, Texas, where he set up a clinic for treating internal cancer. At its peak, the clinic had ten thousand patients on its books, charging each one a fixed four hundred dollar fee, prescribing a "pink medicine" and a "black medicine." The former contained lactated pepsin and potassium iodide, the latter a botanical laxative in an extract of prickly ash bark, buckthorn bark, barberry root, licorice root, pokeweed, alfalfa, and red clover blossoms (32, 179).

Third, two Yugoslavian brothers named Durovic brought from Argentina to the United States a whitish powder called Krebiozen, said to have come from the blood of horses which had been injected with a micro-organism responsible for "lumpy jaw" in cattle (179, 180). Their assertion that Krebiozen could cure cancer won the dogged allegiance of one of the nation's leading cancer experts, Dr. Andrew Ivy of the University of Illinois. Thousands of physicians secured vials of this so-called investigational drug for eager patients, making a nine dollar "donation" for each ampul. In 1963 a team of FDA chemists, analyzing the only sample of Krebiozen ever secured from its sponsor, discovered it to be the common amino acid, creatin monohydrate. Simultaneous analyses of the Krebiozen distributed to physicians revealed it to be nothing but mineral oil.

The fourth major promotion has been that of Laetrile.

Laetrile possesses a more complex chronicle and a more varied cast of characters than those of Glyoxilide, Hoxsey's botanicals, and Krebiozen, and has created greater public impact and gained more political power than did its three predecessors. Nonetheless, Laetrile impresses the historian as conforming to a ten-point profile of health quackery derived from a study of past quackish ventures (181).

Exploitation of Fear

Quacks have traditionally scared their victims with disturbing language, frightening pictures, and grim statistics, stressing pain and threat of death. A turn-of-the-century pamphlet described gruesomely how cancer ate away the sufferer's nose, face, palate, and throat (182).

The modern promotional mode employs greater subtlety in playing on the morbid fear of cancer in our society. Laetrile agents try to reach patients when cancer has just been diagnosed and panic is high, and, like others before them, interpret orthodox therapies as essentially useless and more painful than the disease itself. One physician testifying in Kansas City told of a patient who, within a day of having lung cancer diagnosed, received Laetrile advertising in the mail (183). "Cutting, burning, and poisoning" to characterize surgery, radiation, and chemotherapy have become a litany in Laetrile literature (184). "Voodoo witchcraft" would do more good.

Promise of Painless Treatment and Good Results

"No knife or pain," advertised a Chicago cancer quack
in 1912, promising to cure breast cancer (185). The history
of cancer quackery reveals constant assurances of easy treatment and good results. In earlier days, sure cures were
promised. More recently, prudence has dictated greater cau-
tion. By treating cancer with nothing more painful than injections of a non-toxic drug, according to a Laetrile tract,
fifteen percent of patients with advanced metastasized
cancer and eighty percent of those with early diagnosed
cancer "will be saved" (186). And Dr. Richardson evoked
the vision of a cancerless nation in a mere two-score years,
achieved by nothing more arduous than regular oral doses of
Laetrile (107).

Claims of a Miraculous Scientific Breakthrough

Marvelous new discoveries are a dime a dozen in the
literature of quack promotions. In earlier times the secret
might be an herb brought back by a missionary from some primitive overseas tribe or pried loose by an explorer from an
Indian medicine man (187). Hoxsey attributed his botanical
formula to the perception of his great-grandfather who noted
the healing of the cancer on the leg of his horse which
grazed in a pasture where the plants grew (32). Recent
"discoveries" have generally been said to derive from in-
spired research. The Durovics' horse experiments in the
Argentine furnish an example.

Laetrile's heroic tale centers on the humble physician,
Ernst Krebs, Sr., busy with his practice yet always seeking
out drugs and vitamins to benefit mankind, and on his son,
Krebs, Jr., inveterate researcher, who modified the cyanide-
containing chemical his father had found in apricot kernels
so that it could kill cancer cells but leave healthy cells
unharmed (2). To the audiences at the legion of Laetrile
meetings before which Krebs, Jr., appears, he has become a
figure of awe and veneration, acclaimed as a Pasteur and
linked with the signers of the Declaration of Independence
(188), a myth in his own time.

One Cause/One Therapeutic System

Quacks often win allegiance to their doctrines by
promising to end confusion and doubt and to make complexity
simple and comprehensible to the untutored mind. Disease,
the quack says, has but one cause. Therefore, one treatment
is all that is needed to fight it. In the nineteenth century Benjamin Brandreth blamed all illness on vitiation of

the blood caused by constipation (189). For a perfect panacea, therefore, try Brandreth's cathartic pills. Later
Samuel Hartman's high-alcoholic Peruna promised only to cure
catarrh, but Hartman defined catarrh to cover almost every
symptom in the book (190).

A similar sweeping boldness has operated in the cancer
realm. Reputable authorities now assert that there are as
many different cancers as there are different common colds,
over a hundred, with a broad range of causes. But for Koch
all cancer came from a single toxin. For Hoxsey all cancer
resulted from a disturbance in body chemistry. At the start,
Laetrile's sponsors rooted their explanation in the unitarian or trophoblastic theory, and more lately have denominated
all cancer dietary deficiency disease. Initially Laetrile
alone played the role of virtual specific. "Laetrile does
not palliate," Dr. Krebs wrote in an early pamphlet, "it
acts chemically to kill the cancer cell selectively without
injury to the normal tissues of the body" (191). Recently
Laetrile in its new guise of Vitamin B-17 has assumed central
place in a therapeutic system, complex, but according to its
proponents, integrated. Robert Bradford envisioned metabolic
health centers as "the wave of the medical future," replac-
ing orthodoxy's rugged and allegedly futile methods, and
heralding the day "when the killer degenerative [disease]
. . . of the civilized world would come to an end" (150).
In the same year Dr. John Richardson could posit use of
Laetrile alone as a universal cancer preventive (107).

The implication of these futuristic claims is bold
enough, in contrast with the restraint about Laetrile's
current effectiveness in public utterances. At the hearings
held by the FDA in Kansas City and by Senator Kennedy's
subcommittee in Washington, Laetrile's sponsors made the
most modest of claims. The public record, however, and
private conversations sometimes take on a different tone.
Ernst Krebs, Jr., could say in Kansas City, "We disclaim
saving anyone's life" (60). But during a trial at which the
state of California had charged Krebs with violating his probation, evidence indicated that his promises were not so
circumscribed (192). A widow testified that her husband,
learning that he had lung cancer, had rejected the operation
which his doctor had told him had a ninety percent chance of
success. Instead, having heard Krebs on television, the man
looked his name up in the telephone directory and asked his
advice. Krebs told the inquirer that, if he relied on Laetrile, his chance of recovery would be one hundred percent.
Krebs sent the man to Dr. Richardson. Nine months later the
man was dead.

The Galileo Ploy

In response to criticism from the community of scientists, quackery has often brought into play the Galileo ploy. The unorthodox say the orthodox are wrong, just as earlier critics condemned pioneering explorers, inventors, and scientists. We are, the unorthodox assert, like Columbus, Jenner, and Pasteur -- the list is long. We are today misunderstood by blind men but are destined to be heroes to future generations.

In 1951 at the trial of a woman who sold a so-called Radio Therapeutic Instrument, claiming it could cure cancer of the breast with rays beamed over great distances, her attorney trotted out Columbus, Harvey, and Semmelweiss in her defense (193). Laetrile promoters have offered the same gambit. The text of a film strip, World Without Cancer, likened Krebs, Jr., to these three worthies, as well as to Galileo and the Wright brothers (184). In praising Krebs before Senator Kennedy's subcommittee, Robert Bradford admitted that Krebs had "only an honorary doctorate," then added: "Are you aware, gentlemen, that Christopher Columbus never went to nautical school? Can we recall the shoddy credentials of Thomas Edison? Was Albert Einstein all that bright a student in school?" (95).

The Conspiracy Theory

Another time-tested response to criticism is the shouting of conspiracy. The scientific establishment doesn't dare recognize the validity of my great discovery, the quack claims, for it will undermine their power and prestige and eliminate their jobs. So the establishment scientists conspire to suppress the wonderful new remedy.

Koch, Hoxsey, and the Krebiozen forces all resorted to the conspiracy theory, and so do the Laetrile supporters. Dr. Richardson sees the Rockefeller family at the center of the web, controlling pharmaceutical manufacturers and preventing them from developing drugs not made from oil (194). The Rockefellers also control the American Cancer Society, a staunch foe of Laetrile. In this nightmare, the National Cancer Institute, the Food and Drug Administration, and organized medicine are likewise deemed members of the selfish conspiracy to suppress Laetrile.

Shifts to Adjust to Circumstances

Quackery has never felt obliged to retain a given posture if some change might offer greater prosperity or safety.

In the nineteenth century a cold cure that wasn't selling
became a stomach remedy and reaped huge profits.

Laetrile's history has been marked by many changes.
When the Krebs' version of amygdalin emerged, chemotherapy
as a mode of treating cancer was new, public excitement
about it high. The first pro-Laetrile paperback, Kittler's
Control for Cancer, grafted the apricot pit drug onto that
interest, stressed Laetrile's chemical nature, did not mention the word "vitamin" (2). By the 1970s nature's way
toward health enjoyed great public favor, chemicals in cancer
therapy had slipped some in popular prestige, and chemicals
in the environment had come under grave suspicion. John
Richardson's Laetrile Case Histories blasted chemotherapy in
cancer, denied explicitly that Laetrile was a "drug," and
concluded that control of cancer had been found "in nature"
(195). From drug to vitamin, from cure to palliative and
preventive, from low dosage to high dosage level, the pattern
of Laetrile's postures has been kaleidoscopic. "The mere
fact that there is a constantly changing set of theories as
to why laetrile should be used or how it does work,"
asserted the American Medical Association to the Kennedy
subcommittee, "is sufficient to lead objective persons to
question the validity of any of the theories put forth" (196).

Reliance on Testimonials

Through history the testimonial has been a major weapon
in the arsenal of quackery. When someone just like you and
me says, with urgent sincerity, "I was cured," the persuasive
power ranks high. "Our experience of more than thirty years
in the enforcement of the Food and Drug Act," a former
Commissioner once wrote, "has demonstrated that testimonials
may be obtained for practically any article labeled as a
treatment for practically any disease" (197). But testimonials given in the first flush of hope prove sadly premature. Old newspapers contain instances of testimonials
appearing in the same issues with the obituaries of the
testators (198). Modern science holds that drug efficacy
can not be determined by individual instances, nor even by a
series of such cases. Much more sophisticated scientific
methods are required. As a matter of law, the Supreme Court
has so ruled (199).

All major cancer unorthodoxies have relied heavily on
testimonials. The despairing cancer victim hears or reads
such success stories as part of an enthusiastic promotional
presentation, one that resounds with a sense of conviction
and with every evidence of sincere concern for the victim's
welfare. He is offered hope, told things he himself may do

to take his own treatment into his own hands. His new painless therapy, his new diet, his sense of support from new
acquaintances, his more cheerful expectations, do indeed
enhance the way he feels. The placebo effect is powerful,
if temporary, medicine. An injection of confidence may indeed give the patient a better appetite, let him gain weight,
enhance the way he looks, improve the way he feels. If he
has been suffering from the side effects of effective treatment, perhaps nausea and the loss of hair, a switch to unorthodoxy may end these unpleasant consequences. Under
these circumstances both the patient and the doctor who is
administering the unorthodox treatment may pen testimonials.
If, as a result of previous or concomitant orthodox therapy,
the patient's health may indeed be improved, the testimonial
may nonetheless give all the credit to unorthodoxy.

In preparing for legal action against Hoxsey's enterprise, the Food and Drug Administration investigated the
writers of all the testimonials which Hoxsey had printed in
behalf of his internal cancer treatment (32). Hoxsey's
claimed cures, the FDA was able to demonstrate in court, fell
into three classes. Either the patients had never had cancer
-- and some cancers are extremely difficult to diagnose --
although treated for it at Hoxsey's Dallas clinic. Or they
had been cured of cancer by proper orthodox treatment before
or while consulting Hoxsey. Or they had had cancer and
either still were afflicted despite Hoxsey's treatment or
else had died. This evidence substantiated the scientific
inadequacy of anecdotal evidence, no matter how sincere the
testimony. The same findings resulted from the National
Cancer Institute's evaluation of Dr. Contreras' cases (166).

Further, one of the odd paradoxes relating to quackery
is that failure seldom diminishes patient loyalty. The
duped seem unable to realize deception has occurred. The
quack has done such a good job of exuding sincerity and concern that the victim believes the false explanation that
the specious remedy or routine would have healed had treatment only begun a little sooner. And the misery of the
decline toward death had seemed, under the unorthodox regimen, less arduous than would otherwise have been the case
(200).

Laetrile promotion has relied heavily on testimonial
evidence, given by patients before legislative committees,
compiled by Laetrile advocates between the covers of books.
The scientific weakness of such an approach, as exemplified
by Dr. John Richardson's Laetrile Case Histories, receives
stark underlining in the analysis of this volume presented
in Commissioner Kennedy's report to the Oklahoma court (21).

Distortion of the Idea of "Freedom"

Before food and drug laws were enacted, quacks waved
the banner of "freedom" to smear criticism aimed at them by
physicians and pharmacists. When drug laws came, quacks
formed protest groups with high-sounding names, like the
National League for Medical Freedom and the American Medical
Liberty League (201). "Freedom" is certainly one of the
most treasured words in the American lexicon. As has been
seen above, the manipulation of this word by unorthodox
health promoters has constituted their major symbolic campaign during the last quarter century. Thus Laetrile's
loud appeal for "freedom of choice" in cancer therapy is
nothing new. Pushed with vigor, however, by those with
untraconservative convictions about the governmental role in
society, in a climate of opinion worried about over-regula-
tion, Laetrile's "freedom" pitch has persuaded more numerous
converts to its cause than any previous unorthodoxy has
succeeded in winning. The prevailing mythology of cancer,
Susan Sontag has written, conjoins with "a simplistic view
of the world that can turn paranoid." "Perhaps," she adds,
"right-wing groups are the main organized support for quack
cures like Laetrile because they also share a paranoid view
of the world" (178).

Such a direction for "freedom" leads toward the license
of those ancient days, when "the toadstool millionaires,"
operating without restraint, fleeced and often killed their
victims. That is a fate from which seven decades of con-
structive legislation, beginning with the Pure Food and Drugs
Act of 1906, has somewhat rescued the nation. Complex,
modern, industrial, urbanized society, with standards of
medical judgment far more precise than in the nineteenth
century, can not afford to let the nation's health concerns
be governed by a distorted definition of that great symbol
"freedom" which would return piratical anarchy to the realm
of health.

Large Sums of Money Are Involved

It was Oliver Wendell Holmes who termed nineteenth century nostrum vendors "toadstool millionaires" (202). They
might not make a million, but money was their goal.

Laetrile is big business. Investigations by California
authorities revealed what huge sums some of the Laetrile
leaders had been putting in the bank (36, 92). Robert
Bradford, according to an agent of the Food and Drug Bureau

cited in the New York Times, had been taking in an estimated
$150,000 to $200,000 a month in Laetrile sales. In slightly
over two years, Dr. John Richardson had deposited some
$2,800,000 in a single checking account (203). The quantity
of Laetrile that Judge Bohanon determined to be a six-month
supply would have cost the user about $2250 (204). Estimating
Laetrile users at 75,000, the mathematics mounts to millions.

Laetrile Within the Perspective of the Past

Fear of cancer, suspicion of government, a primitivis-
tic retreat from complex civilization to "natural" ways,
skillful organization, adept lobbying, and a shrewdness at
borrowing time-tested techniques from quackery's well-
stocked past, such factors undergird the Laetrile movement.
In the face of scientific evidence and informed advice,
frightened people place vain hope in it.

What guide might the past provide as to Laetrile's
future? The other major cancer unorthodoxies of the twentieth century, Glyoxilide, Hoxsey's botanicals, Krebiozen,
have virtually disappeared within the United States, although they linger outside the nation's borders, available
to the desperate traveler. What brought Koch, Hoxsey, the
Durovics and Ivy down from their peaks of prominence was a
combination of vigorous regulatory action, sustained
critique, and faddist fascination with still newer unorthodoxies.

Dr. William Koch underwent two very long trials in 1943
and 1946, charged with promoting misbranded and ineffective
drugs (179). The first ended with a hung jury, the second
when a juror became ill. Koch gave up business and retired
to Brazil. Against Harry Hoxsey, the Food and Drug Administration initiated numerous actions. Injunction proceedings
begun in 1950 before a judge disposed in Hoxsey's favor were
finally won only after the case had twice reached the Supreme
Court (32). In 1957 an injunction closed Hoxsey's satellite
operation in Pennsylvania. Krebiozen came to a halt in interstate commerce when its sponsors withdrew a plan for the investigational use of the drug which they had submitted to the
FDA (179, 180). This ban held, even though the government
failed to convict the Durovics and Dr. Ivy in a nine-month
criminal case decided in 1966 by a Chicago jury. Later, an
investigation of jury tampering led to the conviction and
jailing of one of the jurors. Thus regulatory action almost
completely removed the unorthodox cancer treatments from
interstate commerce, permitting their sponsors almost no elbow
room for continuing promotion.

Not that unorthodoxy did not fight back. Hoxsey, for
example, strove strenuously for political support, gaining
favorable recognition from several United States Senators
(32). And he sought to establish and ally with organized
support for his cancer clinic. In 1959 Hoxsey spoke at a
naturopathic convention in Chicago, which also hearkened to
the National Health Federation's president, Fred J. Hart.
At NHF membership rallies, Hart solicited funds to help
Hoxsey carry on his contest with the FDA, and Hoxsey in turn
gave royalties from his autobiography to help finance the
NHF. Despite his efforts, Hoxsey did not develop an institutional base broad and strong enough to permit his unorthodox clinics to survive. Nor did the promoters of Glyoxilide
or Krebiozen succeed with similar attempts.

Prior to Laetrile's series of victories in the legislatures of seventeen states, the major political triumph
achieved by the forces of unorthodoxy came in the national
Congress with the enactment of the Vitamin Amendments of
1976 (102). Led by the National Health Federation, promoters of nutritional products skillfully mobilized their
followers into a powerful lobbying force. By securing the
new law, the health food industry not only succeeded in
thwarting the Food and Drug Administration's attempt to
tighten the stringency of regulation in this field, they won
from Congress a curtailment of FDA's authority below that
which had been given the agency by Congress in the 1938 law.

This episode reveals that health unorthodoxy has the
capability of mounting sufficient political power to win
important victories. The obviously growing strength of
nutritional unorthodoxy may well have played a role in
Laetrile's transmogrification into a "vitamin." The National
Health Federation has accepted and promoted Laetrile's
vitamin status. In 1977 the NHF made legalizing Laetrile
its "No. 1 priority" (205). It remains to be seen whether
the millions of Americans who flirt with nutritional unorthodoxy will welcome an anti-cancer Vitamin B-17. Not all
citizens who believe in extra vitamins as a sure road to
extra pep may so readily accept vitamins in the treatment of
cancer.

No previous cancer unorthodoxy ever approximated the
institutional base which Laetrile achieved, resting on the
International Association of Cancer Victims and Friends; the
Cancer Control Society, formed by dissident members of the
IACVF (206); and particularly the Committee for Freedom of
Choice in Cancer Therapy, whose motivation is as much poli-
tical as therapeutic. The big question is whether this poli-
tical base is firm enough to establish Laetrile in an

institutionalized sense in our society, whatever else may
happen. Indeed, it may be surmised that Laetrile's boom
has peaked and now is in decline. Reports about toxicity
doubtless dampened public ardor. Laetrile bills before
state legislatures did not fare so well during 1978 as in
1977 (115). Future consideration and reconsideration may
find state assemblymen looking more probingly past the
freedom of choice argument at the scientific facts, following the example of Massachusetts (207). Inquiries about
Laetrile to the Food and Drug Administration have fallen off
(208). Media coverage has declined, despite such newsworthy
events as the announcement of the National Cancer Institute's
proposed trials and the Tenth Circuit's decision in the
Rutherford case. Even should that decision stand, the legal
use of Laetrile would be drastically curtailed from the
level defined in Judge Bohanon's decision, with oral dosage
forms eliminated. The Supreme Court, in adjudicating between
the Tenth and Seventh Circuits, may confirm the FDA's
authority to ban Laetrile completely from interstate commerce (209).

     Even if Laetrile should follow Krebiozen and the others
off center stage, this does not mean unorthodoxy's demise.
As long as cancers remain a grave problem and wear a fearful
image, quackery threatens. Much disenchantment exists with
scientific medicine. Cancer patients have felt rejected by
some orthodox physicians who have seemed to lose interest
in their cases when nothing more medically could be done.
The unorthodox offer considerable psychological support.
The quixotic state of public feelings about health conduces
to strange enthusiasms and open sesame for charlatans.
Despite such a hopeful development as the hospice movement
(210), offering skilled and considerate support to the dying
and their families, a gloomy prognosis is hard to avoid.
The broader and more diffuse approach of metabolic therapy,
in which Laetrile is now enveloped, may prove a more difficult regulatory problem to confront than combatting a single
unproven entity.

     A shrewd and seasoned observer, looking ahead, recently
took a somber tone (211): "During the past decade, a
change has taken place in public attitudes toward medical
science. There has been an increasing acceptance of misin-
formation, as shown for example by the success of the
laetrile and 'health food' movements. This acceptance has
been aided by the media, especially television, which pub-
licize sensational and erroneous statements. These are
seldom rebutted. There is distrust of the 'establishment,'
and a feeling that doctors are exploiting patients. I believe this trend is so well established, and so little

challenged, that its impact will produce a decline of scientific medicine, and its replacement by quackery."

References and Notes

1. Report by Jack Forbragd and Kenneth B. Ewing of interview with Ernst T. Krebs, Sr., Dec. 11, 1962, San Francisco District File CF: 10 183, Krebs Laboratories, vol. 1, Food and Drug Administration Records (San Francisco).
2. G. D. Kittler, Control for Cancer (Paperback Library, New York, 1963).
3. Bull. Nev. State Bd. of Health, Jan. 1920, clipping, FDA report, Dec. 9, 1957, San Francisco District File, CF: 10 183, John Beard Memorial Foundation, vol. 4, FDA Records (San Francisco).
4. Nevada Appeal, Carson City, Nov. 14, 1957, clipping, ibid.
5. Bureau of Chemistry, Department of Agriculture, Notices of Judgment 11193 (1923) and 12047 (1924).
6. FDA D.N.J. 17066 (1930).
7. S. B. Gilmore and J. B. Corson to San Francisco District, Apr. 1, 1958, San Francisco District File, CF: 10 183, John Beard Memorial Foundation, vol. 6, FDA Records (San Francisco).
8. San Francisco District Summary and Recommendation for Prosecution, Oct. 20, 1960, ibid.
9. E. Krebs, Jr., E. Krebs, Sr., and H. H. Beard, The Unitarian or Trophoblastic Thesis of Cancer (McNaughton Foundation, Montreal, 1950).
10. Walter Van Winkle, Jr., to Ernst T. Krebs, May 7, 1945, [re NDA 5703], AF 26-731, vol. 1, FDA Records (Rockville).
11. Edward V. O'Gara to San Francisco District, July 14, 1945, ibid.
12. D. Rorvik, New West, Apr. 25, 1977, p. 51.
13. Affidavit of Ernst T. Krebs, Sr., Apr. 28, 1965, FDA File on Labeling and Composition of Laetrile, FDA Records (Rockville).
14. Statement of Eric E. Conn on Patent Specifications 13228, vol. M, item 424, FDA Administrative Record, Laetrile, Docket No. 77N-0048.
15. Russell C. White and Donald L. Taylor to San Francisco District, Dec. 15, 1952, FDA File on Labeling and Composition of Laetrile, FDA Records (Rockville).
16. Statement of Carol M. Hehmeyer, Banning of the Drug Laetrile from Interstate Commerce by FDA (95th Cong., 1st ses., Hearing before the Subcommittee on Health and Scientific Research of the Committee on Human Resources, U.S. Senate, July 12, 1977 [hereafter, Hearing before Kennedy subcommittee]), pp. 239-40.
17. Ralph Weilerstein to San Francisco District, series of

1945 memoranda, AF 26-731, vol. 1, FDA Records (Rock-ville).

18. Eugene Eno to San Francisco District, Sep. 13, 1950, San Francisco District File, CF: 10 183, John Beard Memorial Foundation, vol. 1, FDA Records (San Francisco).
19. *Science*, 103, 25, (1946).
20. E. T. Krebs, M.D., *Laetrile* (San Francisco, n.d.), in Laetrile file of exhibits, AF 26-731, Accession 88-73-6, box 50, FDA Records, Record Group 88, Washington National Records Center (Suitland, MD) (hereafter, WNRC).
21. FDA, Laetrile, Commissioner's Decision on Status, *Fed. Reg.* 42, 39773 (1977).
22. Richard M. Stalvey to San Francisco District, Sep. 10, 1953, San Francisco District File, CF: 10 183, John Beard Memorial Foundation, vol. 1, FDA Records (San Francisco).
23. Krebs, Jr., to Ian McDonald, Dec. 8, 1952, ibid.
24. Memorandum of interview between Ralph Weilerstein and L. Henry Garland, Dec. 9, 1952, ibid.
25. Cancer Commission of the California Medical Association, *Calif. Med.* 78, 320 (1953).
26. R. T. Dorr and J. Paxinos, *Ann. Internal Med.* 89, 389 (1978).
27. Memorandum of interview between Ralph Weilerstein and E. W. DeLong, Aug. 24, 1953, San Francisco District File, CF: 10 183, John Beard Memorial Foundation, vol. 1, FDA Records (San Francisco).
28. *San Francisco News*, Mar. 24, 1953.
29. Krebs, Jr., to Richard E. Sponholz, Mar. 28, 1961, in Laetrile file of exhibits, AF 26-731, Acc. 88-73-6, box 50, FDA Records, RG 88, WNRC.
30. Patent Specification 788,855 (1958).
31. San Francisco District Report, Dec. 9, 1957, San Francisco District File, CF: 10 183, John Beard Memorial Foundation, vol. 4, FDA Records (San Francisco).
32. J. H. Young, *The Medical Messiahs* (Princeton University Press, Princeton, 1967), pp. 360-89.
33. FDA D.D.N.J. 6543 (1960).
34. M. L. Yakowitz to J. R. Cain, July 6, 1953, AF 26-731, vol. 1. FDA Records (Rockville).
35. Deposition of Andrew R. L. McNaughton, June 2, 1964, *The Canadian Laetrile (Anti-Cancer Drug) Case* (Montreal, 1964), in Laetrile file of exhibits, AF 26-731, Acc. 88-73-6, box 50, FDA Records, RG 88, WNRC.
36. *New York Times*, June 26, 1977.
37. *Newsweek*, June 27, 1977, pp. 48-56.
38. *The Financial Post*, Toronto, Mar. 10, 1973.
39. *SEC* v. *Biozymes International Ltd.*, et al. U.S. District Court, Northern District of California, Civil Action No. C72-2217-SW, Apr. 27, 1973.

40. Memorandum of interview at HEW by W. B. Rankin, Oct. 18, 1961, San Francisco District File, CF: 10 183, John Beard Memorial Foundation, vol. 4, FDA Records (San Francisco).
41. Memorandum of interview at FDA by Ralph G. Smith, Oct. 18, 1961, ibid.
42. FDA D.D.N.J. 7062 (1962).
43. Many documents dealing with the circumstances of Krebs' probation are filed in San Francisco District File 1-412P, vols. 3 and 4, FDA Records (San Francisco).
44. Krebs argued that his violation of the law had been technical, cued by his haste to beat the Russians in pangamic acid research, which, because oxygen utilization was involved, might help the United States triumph over the Soviet Union in the space race. Krebs to Robert M. Ensign, Sep. 18, 1963, ibid., vol. 4.
45. Maurice P. Kerr to Chief Inspector, Dec. 9, 1963, San Francisco District File, CF: 10 183, Krebs Laboratories, vol. 1, FDA Records (San Francisco).
46. Krebs to John A. Sprague, May 1, 1963, San Francisco District File 1-412P, vol. 3, FDA Records (San Francisco).
47. Gregory S. Stout to California State Board of Health, June 27, 1963, ibid., vol. 4.
48. G. D. Kittler, "The Struggle," *American Weekly*, Mar. 3 and 10, 1963.
49. James Nakada to District Directors, May 1, 1963, San Francisco District File 1-412P, vol. 3, FDA Records, (San Francisco).
50. Interview with Cecile Pollack Hoffman by William P. Leckwold, Feb. 12, 1965, San Francisco District File, CF: 10 183, Krebs Laboratories, vol. 1, FDA Records (San Francisco).
51. McKay McKinnon to Wallace Janssen, June 12, 1964, San Francisco District File 1-412P, vol. 4, FDA Records, (San Francisco).
52. Arthur Dickerman to William Goodrich, Jan. 25, 1963, ibid., vol. 3.
53. Memorandum of interview with McNaughton by G. S. Goldhammer, Feb. 1, 1963, ibid.
54. California Cancer Advisory Council, *Report on the Treatment of Cancer with Beta-Cyanogenetic Gluosides (Laetriles)* (1963), exhibit to affidavit of W. Sherwood Lawrence, Vol. F, item 183, FDA Administrative Record, Laetrile, Docket No. 77N-0048.
55. *San Francisco Examiner*, June 6, 1963.
56. *FDA Report on Enforcement and Compliance*, Aug. 1964, pp. 8-9.
57. William C. Hill to K. F. Ernst, May 25, 1967, Krebs Injunction 508 File, vol. 2, FDA Records (San Francisco).

58. San Francisco District Report, Sep. 22, 1969, San Francisco District File, CF: 10 183, Krebs Laboratories, vol. for 1969-71, FDA Records (San Francisco).

59. San Francisco Chronicle, Jan. 27, 1970.

60. Testimony of Ernst Krebs, Jr., vol. O-1, FDA Administrative Record, Laetrile, Docket No. 77N-0048.

61. Numerous documents during 1969 and 1970 in San Francisco District File, CF: 10 183, Krebs Laboratories, FDA Records (San Francisco).

62. FDA news release about NDA 6734, Sep. 1, 1971.

63. HEW Secretary Elliot Richardson to Congressman Lawrence H. Fountain, Aug. 26, 1971, AF 26-731, vol. 12, FDA Records (Rockville).

64. FDA letters to McNaughton Foundation, Apr. 20 and 28, 1970, ibid.

65. Don C. Matchan in Alameda (CA) Times-Star, July 14, 1970.

66. Dean Burk to Secretary Richardson, Mar. 23, 1971, AF 26-731, vol. 12, FDA Records (Rockville).

67. Dean Burk, in Who's Who in America, 40th Edition, 1978-1979 (Marquis Who's Who, Chicago, 1978), vol. 1, p. 470.

68. C. P. Hoffman and E. N. Blaauw, If It Is True Cancer Can Be Controlled Why Isn't It?, 1964 pamphlet, in San Francisco District File, CF: 10 183, Krebs Laboratories, vol. 1, FDA Records (San Francisco).

69. James A. Crandall to Los Angeles District, July 12, 1965, ibid., vol. for 1965-68.

70. John W. Holten to Los Angeles District, Aug. 23, 1965, ibid.

71. Memorandum of telephone conversation between Gordon R. Wood and T. M. Rice, June 23, 1969, ibid., vol. for 1969-71.

72. S. Barrett and G. Knight, eds., The Health Robbers (George F. Stickley, Philadelphia, 1976), p. 9.

73. Ibid., pp. 189-201.

74. Young, The Medical Messiahs, pp. 383-84, 400-401.

75. Clippings from the National Health Federation Bulletin, Prevention, and National Enquirer, AF 26-731, vol. 11, FDA Records (Rockville).

76. Walter Ermer to M. J. Ryan, Oct. 16, 1970, ibid.

77. Numerous letters, ibid., vols. 11 and 12.

78. NHF Bulletin, Sep. 1970, clipping, ibid., vol. 11.

79. Fountain to Richardson, Mar. 16, 1971, ibid., vol. 12.

80. FDA news release, Sep. 1, 1971, with attached Report of the Ad Hoc Committee of Oncology Consultants.

81. H. R. 12092, introduced by John G. Schmitz, Dec. 7, 1971, Cong. Rec., 92nd Cong., 1st ses., p. 45120.

82. People v. Ernst T. Krebs, Jr., Malvina Cassese, and Byron

Krebs, San Francisco Municipal Court, Dept. 6, Docket No. G-14656 et al.

83. Testimony of Carol M. Hehmeyer, Hearing before Kennedy subcommittee, pp. 226, 237.

84. Resume of Laetrile cases, State of California, Health and Welfare Agency, Department of Health Services, various dates.

85. People v. Mary Whelchel, San Diego Superior Court, Dept. 18, Docket CR 23718, Jan. 14 and 17, 1972; Feb. 13, 1974.

86. Her Majesty the Queen v. Andrew R. L. McNaughton, Province of Quebec, District of Montreal, Court of Sessions of the Peace, No. 499-72, Judgment, Apr. 22, 1974.

87. McNaughton pleaded guilty to a charge of conspiracy to facilitate the transportation of smuggled Laetrile. United States v. Andrew R. L. McNaughton, U.S. District Court, Southern District of California, No. 76-0448-Criminal, Judgment, Dec. 12, 1977.

88. Newsday, Apr. 23, 1977.

89. Unsigned memorandum for file, Mar. 10, 1972, AF 26-731, vol. 19, FDA Records (Rockville).

90. J. A. Richardson and P. Griffin, Laetrile Case Histories (Bantam Books, New York, 1977), pp. 13-17, 71-73.

91. California Board of Medical Quality Action Report, 10/1/76-12/30/76, John A. Richardson, M.D., Albany, Nov. 29, 1976.

92. Testimony of Herbert B. Hoffman, Joseph Consentino, and Louis Castro, Hearing before Kennedy subcommittee, pp. 189-98.

93. Robert W. Bradford to Dear Friend, The Committee for Freedom of Choice in Cancer Therapy brochure, [early 1973], in AF 26-731, vol. 22, FDA Records (Rockville).

94. San Francisco Chronicle, Aug. 11, 1976.

95. Statement of Robert W. Bradford, Hearing before Kennedy subcommittee, pp. 280-311.

96. Affidavit of O. E. Kelly, vol. K, item 389, FDA Administrative Record, Laetrile, Docket No. 77N-0048.

97. U.S. v. Bradford and U.S. v. Richardson, U.S. District Court, Southern District, California, 76-0448 Criminal, Judgment and Probation filed Dec. 12, 1977; U.S. v. Richardson, Bowman, Salaman, and Bradford, U.S. Court of Appeals, 9th Circuit, Nos. 77-2203, 77-204, 22-2262, and 77-2288, opinion filed Oct. 20, 1978.

98. Ernst Krebs, Sr., to FDA, Apr. 18, 1963, San Francisco District File, CF: 10 183, John Beard Memorial Foundation, vol. 6, FDA Reocrds (San Francisco).

99. E. T. Krebs, Jr., Jnl. Applied Nutrition 22, 75 (1970).

100. Frank D. Corum memorandum, Mar. 24, 1966, San Francisco District File 131-699B, FDA Records (San Francisco).

101. National Analysts, Inc., A Study of Health Practices and Opinions (National Technical Information Service, Springfield, VA, 1972).
102. J. H. Young, "The Agile Role of Food," in Nutrition and Drug Interrelations, J. N. Hathcock and J. Coon, eds. (Academic Press, New York, 1978), pp. 1-18.
103. D. M. Greenberg, West. J. Med., 122, 345 (1975).
104. National Nutrition Consortium, Inc., Statement on Laetrile-Vitamin B$_{17}$, Dec. 21, 1976.
105. T. H. Jukes, Nutrition Today 12, 12 (Sep.-Oct. 1977).
106. Testimony of Thomas H. Jukes, vol. 0-1, FDA Administrative Record, Laetrile, Docket No. 77N-0048.
107. Testimony of John A. Richardson, Robert Bradford, Ernst T. Krebs, Jr., and Bruce Halstead, Hearing before Kennedy subcommittee, pp. 272-74.
108. Mercury, San Jose, Sep. 7, 1972.
109. Merlyn Wurscher to San Francisco District, Oct. 19, 1972, San Francisco District File, CF: 10 183, Krebs Laboratories, vol. for 1972, FDA Records (San Francisco).
110. FDA N.J.s 29 (Oct. 1975) and 31 (Nov. 1975).
111. FDA N.J.s 32 and Inj. 660 (Apr. 1978).
112. Sacramento Bee, June 24, 1978. On the California cancer quackery law, first enacted in 1959 and made permanent in 1969, see L. F. Saylor, Calif. Med. 112, 94 (1970).
113. H. R. 12573, introduced by Steven D. Symms, Mar. 16, 1976, 94th Cong. 2nd ses., p. H2002.
114. Symms interview, U. S. News and World Report, June 13, 1977, pp. 51-52.
115. S. L. Nightingale and F. D. Arnold, Legal Aspects of Medicine 6, 31 (1978).
116. Affidavit of Peter H. Wiernik, vol. H. item 200, FDA Administrative Record, Laetrile, Docket No. 77N-0048.
117. New York Times, May 2, Aug. 16 and 25, 1977; June 7, 1978.
118. Atlanta Journal and Constitution, Nov. 20, 1977.
119. Based on author's observations in one state and conversations with several observers in other states.
120. Arizona Republic, Phoenix, June 20, 1977.
121. Chicago Tribune, Aug. 27, 1978.
122. Chicago Sun-Times, Mar. 5, 1978.
123. Rutherford v. United States, 399 F. Supp. 1208 (W.D. Okla., 1975).
124. Medical World News, June 28, 1976, pp. 17-20. Medical World News quotes Rutherford as saying that in Mexico surgeons "cauterized" the growth, and also quotes a Chicago pathologist as stating: "It is exceptionally rare for this type of tumor to metastasize. Local

excision of the polyp virtually always cures the patient."

125. Rutherford v. United States, 542 F. 2d 1137 (10th Cir. 1976).
126. FDA Administrative Record, Laetrile, Docket No. 77N-0048.
127. Rutherford v. United States, 438 F. Supp. 1287 (W. D., Okla. 1977).
128. Rutherford v. United States, 10th Circuit opinion, text cited in United States v. Rutherford, Petition for a Writ of Certiorari, filed with the Supreme Court, Oct. 10, 1978.
129. Statement of Joseph F. Ross, with exhibits, Hearing before Kennedy subcommittee, pp. 62-188.
130. Medical World News, Jan. 9, 1978, pp. 16, 21.
131. Charlotte (NC) Observer, Sep. 12, 1976.
132. P. Lehmann, FDA Consumer 11, 10 (Oct. 1977).
133. F. P. Smith et al., JAMA 238, 1361 (1977).
134. FDA Talk Paper, July 12, 1978.
135. United States v. Mosinee Corp., Inj. 789, FDA news release, May 16, 1977.
136. FDA news release, Aug. 18, 1978.
137. On June 18, 1979, a unanimous Supreme Court reversed the Tenth Circuit, holding that the safety and effectiveness standards in the law do apply to terminal patients. The high court did not address some issues which the district court had raised but the circuit court had not. United States v. Rutherford, No. 78-605.
138. People v. Privitera, Court of Appeals, Fourth Appellate District, Division One, 4 Cr. No. 8323 (1977).
139. The Supreme Court reversed the appellate course in this case. People v. Privitera, Supreme Court of the State of California, No. Crim. 20340 (1979), Sup., 153 Cal. Rptr. 431.
140. Atlanta Constitution, Feb. 1-23, 1978, passim.
141. FDA news release, Mar. 26, 1978.
142. FDA Drug Bulletin, Nov.-Dec. 1977.
143. United States v. Articles of Drug ... Amigdalina Cyto Pharma De Mexico, S.A., Docket No. K77-1283, U.S. District Court for Maryland, filed Aug. 4, 1977, cited in Brief Amicus Curiae of the American Cancer Society, by Grace Powers Monaco, Mar. 8, 1979, in United States v. Rutherford, No. 78-605, in the Supreme Court of the United States, October Term, 1978.
144. Medical World News, Sep. 5, 1977, p. 22.
145. Interview with Eugene Pfeifer, Oct. 25, 1978.
146. On Mar. 31, 1974.
147. Atlanta Constitution, Aug. 21, 1975; Feb. 10, Apr. 1, May 13, 1976; Apr. 19, Dec. 8, 1977; Feb. 9, 1978.

148. American Media, Westlake Village, CA, 1974.
149. '76 Press, Seal Beach, CA, 1976.
150. Choice Publications, Los Altos, CA, 1977.
151. Cited in statement of Robert W. Bradford, Hearing before Kennedy subcommittee, p. 285.
152. Ibid., pp. 272, 310.
153. Los Angeles Times, Sep. 8, 1977.
154. H. W. Manner, The Remission of Tumors with Laetrile Therapy (text of presentation to annual meeting, NHF, 1977).
155. Robert S. K. Young, Review of "The Remission of Tumors with Laetrile Therapy" (text of critique, 1977).
156. M. B. Lipsett and J. C. Fletcher, N. Engl. J. Med. 297, 1183 (1977).
157. F. J. Ingelfinger, N. Eng. J. Med. 296, 1167 (1977). After toxicity evidence concerning Laetrile had begun to mount, Ingelfinger told a reporter that he might not write the kind of editorial again that he had earlier written. Chicago Sun-Times, Mar. 8, 1978.
158. New York Times, Feb. 11, 1977.
159. C. G. Moertel, N. Eng. J. Med. 298, 218 (1978).
160. Statement of Donald Kennedy, Hearing before Kennedy subcommittee, pp. 26-38.
161. Hearing before Kennedy subcommittee, pp. 248-50, 295.
162. Statement by Guy R. Newell, M.D., Deputy Director, National Cancer Institute, on Retrospective Evaluation of Laetrile Anticancer Activity in Man, Jan. 26, 1978.
163. Neil M. Ellison, Report on a Doctors' Workshop on Metabolic Therapy, Amygdalin, and Cancer--Newark, New Jersey, Feb. 4-5, 1978.
164. N. M. Ellison, D. P. Byar and G. R. Newell, N. Engl. J. Med. 299, 549 (1978).
165. Atlanta Constitution, Sep. 28, 1978. In December 1978 the NCI formally applied to the FDA for an IND to permit the clinical trials.
166. Robert C. Wetherell, Jr., Status of Laetrile, Feb. 6, 1975, AF 26-731, vol. 31, FDA Records (Rockville).
167. Newsday, Apr. 25, 1977.
168. Dean Burk to Edward Kennedy, Nov. 16, 1977, and exhibits, Hearing before Kennedy subcommittee, pp. 384-419.
169. Testimony of Robert W. Bradford, vol. 0-2, FDA Administrative Record, Laetrile, Docket No. 77N-0048.
170. D. Leff, Medical World News, May 1, 1978, pp. 43-51.
171. Editorial, The Choice, 4, 2 (Oct. 1978).
172. J. H. Young, Cimarron Rev., No. 8, 31 (1969).
173. New York Times, July 1, 1906.
174. Pennsylvania Gazette, Philadelphia, Oct. 17 and 31, 1745.

175. Young, The Medical Messiahs, pp. 48-49.
176. American Cancer Society, 1977 Cancer Facts & Figures (New York, 1976).
177. Donald Kennedy, text of speech on "Cancer Politics," Nov. 3, 1977.
178. Susan Sontag, New York Review, Jan. 26, pp. 10-16; Feb. 9, pp. 27-29; and Feb. 23, 1978, pp. 29-33. These articles have been combined into a book, Illness as Metaphor (Farrar, Straus and Giroux, New York, 1978).
179. W. F. Janssen, Analytical Chem., 50, 197A (1978).
180. Young, The Medical Messiahs, pp. 401-402, 420.
181. This pattern the author first explored in Newsday, May 1, 1978.
182. American Medical Association, Nostrums and Quackery, 2nd ed. (AMA Press, Chicago, 1912), p. 56.
183. Testimony of David T. Carr, vol. 0-1, FDA Administative Record, Laetrile, Docket No. 77N-0048.
184. G. Edmund Griffin, World Without Cancer, transcript of sound track of documentary film, supplied by Food and Drug Administration.
185. American Medical Association, Nostrums and Quackery, p. 39.
186. G. Edmund Griffin, in Richardson, Laetrile Case Histories, p. 64.
187. J. H. Young, The Toadstool Millionaires (Princeton University Press, Princeton, 1961), pp. 165-89.
188. San Francisco Chronicle, Aug. 11, 1976.
189. Young, Toadstool Millionaires, pp. 75-89.
190. Ibid., pp. 220-21.
191. Affidavit of W. Sherwood Lawrence, vol. F, item 183, FDA Administrative Record, Laetrile, Docket No. 77N-0048.
192. California v. Krebs and Cassese, San Francisco Municipal Court, No. G 14673 and G 14670, 1977.
193. Young, The Medical Messiahs, pp. 239-57.
194. Richardson, Laetrile Case Histories, pp. 97-102.
195. Ibid., pp. xv, 4, 55-65.
196. Statement of the American Medical Association, Hearing before Kennedy subcommittee, pp. 327-32.
197. W. G. Campbell to Leland M. Ford, Mar. 4, 1941, Interstate Office Seizure No. 16224-E File, FDA Records, RG 88, National Archives Branch, WNRC.
198. Arthur J. Cramp, Nostrums and Quackery and Pseudo-Medicine (AMA, Chicago, 1936), pp. 198-208.
199. Weinburger v. Hynson, Westcott & Dunning, Inc., 412 U.S. 609.

200. An apparent example of this circumstance is revealed
     in a letter headed "Cancer and Oncologists versus
     Laetrile," July 25, 1975, AF 26-731, vol. 30, FDA
     Records (Rockville).
201. Cramp, Nostrums and Quackery and Pseudo-Medicine, pp.
     218-21.
202. O. W. Holmes, Medical Essays (Houghton Mifflin, Boston,
     1891), p. 186.
203. Richardson comments on these circumstances in Laetrile
     Case Histories, pp. 76-77.
204. Order and Affidavit and Extension, filed May 10, 1977,
     by Judge Luther Bohanon, Rutherford v. United States.
     I have multiplied the quantity of tablets and inject-
     able liquid authorized by the then current cost, one
     dollar a tablet and ten dollars for a 3g. ampul.
205. Form letter from National Health Federation, [Dec.
     1977], promoting "Fund to Stop Government Ban on
     Laetrile," Decimal File 539.ILX, vol. 33, FDA Records
     (Rockville).
206. A most useful sociological study of persons who attend-
     ed a "Cancer Control Symposium" sponsored by a Michigan
     chapter of the Cancer Control Society appears in G. E.
     Markle, J. C. Petersen, and M. O. Wagenfeld, Soc. Sci.
     & Med., 12, 31 (1978).
207. Boston Herald-American, May 19, 1978.
208. Interview with Stuart L. Nightingale, Oct. 24, 1978.
209. It has been suggested, however, that the right of pri-
     vacy doctrine established by the Supreme Court in
     Griswold v. Connecticut, 381 U. S. 479 (1965), might
     provide grounds for a challenge of federal law restric-
     tions on the consumer's free choice of drugs. D. G.
     Rushing, UCLA Law Rev., 25, 577 (1978).
210. Death Education devoted its double Spring/Summer 1978
     issue to the Hospice movement.
211. Thomas H. Jukes to author, Aug. 11, 1978.

3. Laetrile at Sloan-Kettering: A Case Study

For promising new anti-cancer agents, the traditional route from laboratory to clinic has been via tests in animals. The Food and Drug Administration usually evaluates the suitability of new drugs for testing in human beings on the basis, in part, of the performance of the drugs in appropriate animal models (1). Success in animal tests is thus a prerequisite for clinical trials. But Laetrile, also known as amygdalin or vitamin B-17, has been used by human cancer patients for years, without having been subjected to controlled clinical trials. What data are available about its effects in human cancer patients are largely anecdotal.

There is, however, now a considerable body of literature on the effects of Laetrile on animal tumors, a significant portion of which is derived from experiments conducted at the Sloan-Kettering Institute for Cancer Research in New York City between 1972 and 1977. Like practically every aspect of the scientific and political history of Laetrile, the testing of the compound at Sloan-Kettering has been surrounded by controversy. And despite the fact that the findings of the prestigious research center were predominantly negative in animal studies, the National Cancer Institute has supported going ahead with clinical trials of Laetrile.

Even prior to the extensive Sloan-Kettering experiments with Laetrile, the National Cancer Institute had sponsored a number of studies of the substance in animals (2). These tests had proved to be negative, at least to the satisfaction of their sponsors and the researchers who conducted them. But even though the results of these tests had been widely publicized, they seemed to have had little dampening effect on the use and promotion of Laetrile, nor on calls for clinical tests. In 1972 Benno Schmidt, a member of the board of directors of Sloan-Kettering, called for that institution to test Laetrile thoroughly in animals so that it might be able to back its negative responses to frequent inquiries about the purported cancer cure "with some conviction" (3, p. 1231).

From both a scientific and public relations viewpoint Sloan-Kettering should have been the ideal institution to render a final verdict on Laetrile. Not only was it an internationally known center for research on and treatment of cancer, it also boasted a history of having screened tens of thousands of potential anti-cancer agents in animal tests. The techniques of evaluating new drugs were thus highly developed at the institute. "This institution," said Sloan-Kettering president Lewis Thomas in late 1972, "can answer the Laetrile question fairly quickly" (3, p. 1231).

In addition to the expertise and prestige that Sloan-Kettering promised to bring to its Laetrile experiments, the cancer center studies would also have a technical aspect that would make their results more significant than previous animal tests -- the use of so-called spontaneous tumors.

All previous NCI-sponsored tests had been performed on transplantable animal tumors. As the name implies, these are cancers that develop in one animal and are transferred surgically to another, closely related animal. This technique gives experimenters a high degree of control over the timing, size and site of experimental cancers, but it has been criticized for producing an experimental tumor model that may be quite far removed from the tumors that develop naturally in human patients (4). Spontaneous tumors, by contrast, are those that arise naturally in certain strains of laboratory animals and that are treated in the animal in which they develop, a situation many believe to more closely approximate -- especially in terms of immunological response -- the natural history of many human cancers. The Sloan-Kettering tests, being the first extensive systematic studies of the effects of Laetrile in spontaneous animal tumors, thus promised to be particularly relevant to the question of whether or not clinical trials of Laetrile in human patients might be warranted.

The Sloan-Kettering experiments began under the direction of Lloyd Old, the institute's vice-president for basic research and Chester Stock, the vice-president for chemotherapy research. The initial experiments were carried out by Kanematsu Sugiura, a veteran researcher with more than sixty years experience at the institute.

The material that Sugiura tested was amygdalin prepared in Mexico and supplied to Sloan-Kettering by the McNaughton Foundation, an organization that had been granted and then

quickly denied FDA approval to test Laetrile clinically in
1970. Sugiura used this material to treat a strain of laboratory mice called CD_8F_1, a hybrid in which eighty percent
of the females spontaneously develop mammary tumors at about
the age of ten months.

From the point of view of those who had hoped for a
quick, negative judgment on Laetrile, Sugiura came up with
resoundingly "wrong" results. In three separate experiments
he found that Laetrile, though failing to actually eliminate
the primary tumor, did appear to retard its growth. What's
more, he found that the Laetrile-treated animals had fewer
metastases (secondary tumors) in their lungs than did the
control animals, which received an inert saline solution.
Since it is often the metastatic spread of cancer that is
responsible for the lethal effects of the disease, this finding was of great potential clinical significance. In addition, Sugiura observed that the Laetrile-treated animals
appeared to be livelier and healthier-looking than the control animals.

Sugiura's unexpected findings were not published in the
scientific literature, nor were they made public by Sloan-
Kettering. "If we had published those early positive data,"
Chester Stock later told a journalist, "it would have raised
all kind of havoc" (3). Instead, news of Sugiura's results
was leaked from Sloan-Kettering and publicized by an organization called The Committee for Freedom of Choice in Cancer
Therapy, a pro-Laetrile group founded in 1972 to aid in the
defense of John Richardson, a physician who was being tried
for using Laetrile in cancer therapy. The Committee for
Freedom of Choice is a right-wing group politically, all but
one of its present officers being active members of the
ultra-conservative John Birch Society (5). The Committee
published Sugiura's findings in a pamphlet, "Anatomy of a
Coverup" (6).

Sloan-Kettering's response to Sugiura's results and the
attendant publicity was to step up the Laetrile research
program. Daniel Martin, a surgeon and cancer researcher who
had been supplying the CD_8F_1 mice from his colony at the
Catholic Medical Center in Queens, New York, became an active
participant in the studies. Martin, an outspoken opponent
of Laetrile, conducted independent studies with the substance,
as well as collaborative experiments with Sloan-Kettering
scientists, including Sugiura.

While these additional experiments were being carried
out at Sloan-Kettering and the Catholic Medical Center, the
pro-Laetrile movement was gaining political momentum, achiev-

ing a striking series of political victories. By the middle
of 1977, despite the fact that federal laws still forbade
importation or interstate commerce in Laetrile, the apricot-
pit derivative had received some level of legal acceptance
in more than a dozen states. Even within the medical establishment, the opinion was being voiced that some kind of
clinical evaluation of Laetrile might be desirable, if only
to prove once and for all that it had no worth in the treatment of human cancers. Franz Ingelfinger, then editor of
the New England Journal of Medicine and a cancer patient himself, wrote an editorial calling for the legalized sale and
use of Laetrile. "Prohibition, however," he wrote, "should
be replaced by accurate record-keeping so that patients given
the agent can be identified and followed. Then, after a
period of perhaps two years, an evaluation should be undertaken, not by committees appointed by the FDA or AMA but by
a group broadly representative of society" (7, p. 1168).

It was in this atmosphere of increasing pressure for the
legalization and clinical evaluation of Laetrile that Sloan-
Kettering called a press conference, in June, 1977, to make
public the results of their five years of Laetrile experiments. Reporters attending the conference were given copies
of two scientific papers that were scheduled to appear the
following winter in the Journal of Surgical Oncology. Chester
Stock was the principal author of both papers, one of which
dealt with experiments in transplantable tumors (8) and the
other in spontaneous tumors (9).

The conclusion presented in the two papers, and expressed by Sloan-Kettering spokespersons at the press conference,
was overwhelmingly negative. Laetrile, they reported, had
been confirmed to have no anti-cancer effects against a wide
spectrum of transplantable tumors, and in the spontaneous
systems the verdict was that Laetrile "was found to possess
neither preventive, nor tumor-regressant, nor anti-metastatic,
nor curative anticancer activity" (9).

In none of the collaborative or independent studies conducted after Sugiura's initial positive findings were the
veteran researcher's results duplicated. His findings were
described as "seriously challenged" by the body of subsequent
experiments, including those in which he participated.

Nonetheless it was noted that Sugiura still believed
Laetrile to be a "palliative" if not a cure for cancer, and
when questioned whether he stood by his positive results in
the face of later studies, he responded, "I stick."

As to the question of clinical trials for Laetrile, the

authors of the Sloan-Kettering papers wrote: "We do not have evidence supporting taking amygdalin to clinical trial, although other considerations may require one be conducted" (9).

Among the "other considerations" affecting the future of Laetrile testing was a challenge to the political and scientific integrity of Sloan-Kettering's Laetrile research not from outside or the political right, but from inside and the left. In November of 1977, about five months after the Sloan-Kettering press conference, another press conference was held in New York, this one by a group called Second Opinion, which had just published a 48-page pamphlet on Laetrile at Sloan-Kettering (10). The group charged that the work described in the June Sloan-Kettering papers was "both incomplete and scientifically invalid" (10, p. 1).

The Second Opinion organization described itself as a group of rank-and-file employees of the Memorial Sloan-Kettering Cancer Center, including both scientific and non-scientific personnel. An offshoot of the radical national organization Science For the People, Second Opinion claimed that its basic aim was to organize the workers at Sloan-Kettering. In the "war on cancer," the group advocated "putting prevention first, making research relevant to human diseases," and encouraged "an open-minded policy toward new and unorthodox methods, making the best treatment available to all people, and taking the profit out of cancer"(11, p. 8).

Until the Second Opinion press conference, no employee of Sloan-Kettering had ever publicly identified himself as a member of the organization. The only name openly associated with the group had been that of a City University graduate student. But at this press conference, Ralph Moss, Sloan-Kettering's Assistant Director for Public Affairs, identified himself as a member of Second Opinion. He was fired from that position on the next working day.

According to the Second Opinion report, a fair test of Laetrile had been impossible at Sloan-Kettering from the start. The group's analysis of anti-Laetrile sentiment at the institution included the assertion that Sloan-Kettering had been set up not to produce just any cancer cure, but a patentable one. The pamphlet argued:

> What is wrong is that the promotion of one kind of cancer therapy has brought with it the suppression of other kinds. In this case, a chemical cure for cancer was promoted to the rafters, while most other approaches were ignored or suppressed (10, pp. 46-47).

Though it cited the board of Sloan-Kettering as being made up
of some of "the richest and most powerful men in the world,"
it claimed to "reject all . . . narrow conspiracy theories,
which basically exonerate the real culprit: the profit
system and especially its twentieth century form, monopoly
capitalism" (10, pp. 47-48).

Clearly, the bedfellows made in Laetrile politics proved
to be no less strange than those made in the other political
arenas. Although Second Opinion's press conference was co-
sponsored by the Committee for Freedom of Choice in Cancer
Therapy, Second Opinion specifically stated in its report
that "freedom of choice is not the issue," partly because it
is "not very meaningful to the poor, who cannot afford any
decent cancer treatment, much less private cures in a 'metabolic therapy sanitorium'" (10, p. 48).

The anonymous authors of Second Opinion asked readers of
their report who did not share their political perspective
not to reject their scientific critique of Sloan-Kettering's
Laetrile experiments because of ideological differences.
That critique proved to be a wide-ranging analysis that included charges that Sloan-Kettering had failed to report
pro-Laetrile findings (other than Sugiura's) from experiments
conducted at the center and that it had willfully misrepre-
sented the results of those experiments that it did report.
Most of the criticism was directed toward the crucial studies
of spontaneous tumors. Although Second Opinion claimed to
find some flaws in the experiments with transplantable tumors,
it conceded that the Sloan-Kettering findings in those systems were consistent with those of other researchers and that
in general Laetrile did not seem to be an effective therapeutic agent in such cancers. But in spontaneous tumors the
group claimed that there was "still a need for further examination of amygdalin, as well as related compounds, in spontaneous tumor systems in animals and in man" (10, p. 1).

Among the charges of incompleteness made by Second
Opinion, the most serious was that an experiment had been
carried out between December 1973 and January 1974 in the
laboratory of Elisabeth Stockert at Sloan-Kettering. This experiment was conducted with a strain of laboratory mice that,
like the CD_8F_1 strain with which Sugiura had worked, develops
spontaneous breast cancer. Second Opinion claimed that
Stockert had obtained results similar to those reported by
Sugiura and included in their pamphlet a copy of a memo written by a technician in Stockert's laboratory and addressed to
Sloan-Kettering vice-president Lloyd Old. The technician
reported longer life, healthier appearance, retarded tumor
growth and fewer lung metastases among the mice treated with

Laetrile than among control animals.

Though not challenging the authenticity of the document, Chester Stock explained that his failure to include a report of the experiment in the scientific papers of which he is principal author hardly indicates a will to maliciously "suppress" pro-Laetrile findings. In the first place, he said, he was not even aware of the work until it was brought to his attention by the Second Opinion report. But even had he known about it he insisted that he would never have published it because the results as presented were "uninterpretable" (3, p. 1234). Elisabeth Stockert, in whose laboratory the work was done, attributed the fact that she did not bring the study to Stock's attention to her view of the experiment as only a preliminary study designed not so much to test Laetrile as to familiarize herself and her staff with the animals and material involved. Furthermore, she pointed out that she had been called away to Europe in the middle of the study and that it was therefore never, in her judgment, properly completed (12).

Sloan-Kettering thus acknowledged the existence, though not the validity, of the Stockert experiment. While the version of the paper on experiments with spontaneous tumors presented at the June press conference claimed to present data from "all anti-tumor experiments with amygdalin tested in these spontaneous tumor systems," the version published in the Journal of Surgical Oncology the following spring included the phrase". . . all properly completed anti-tumor experiments. . . ." (13) [underline mine].

Sloan-Kettering never picked up the Second Opinion gauntlet and answered the group's scientific critique on a point by point basis either in the press conference format in which those results were originally presented nor in the less public medium of the scientific literature. The cancer center maintained its initial conclusions about Laetrile and allowed Sugiura's anomalous results to stand unexplained. However, in response to criticisms from within the scientific establishment as well as from Second Opinion, Sloan-Kettering did make one other change in the paper on spontaneous tumors between the June press conference and the Journal of Surgical Oncology publication. The press conference version of the paper contained the following paragraph:

It is concluded that Laetrile (amygdalin) lacks anti-cancer activity against the CD_8F_1 spontaneous mammary tumor. It seems particularly relevant as it is a "solid" tumor with demonstrated clinical therapeutic predictive ability. Of those 8 agents

declared clinically active against human breast
cancer by the National Cancer Institute, all 8
agents also are active against this murine
breast cancer. This unique therapeutic correla-
tion between this animal tumor and human cancer
findings has led to this tumor's selection as
one of the four major animal tumor models of the
national screening program for anti-cancer agents.
Thus, the negative Laetrile findings in this
animal tumor model appear particularly significant
(9).

To many readers this paragraph gave the impression that
Laetrile's failure to show anti-tumor effects in the Sloan-
Kettering tests was an excellent indication that Laetrile
would also fail to work against human cancers because all the
drugs known to work against human breast cancer had been
shown to also work against the spontaneous mouse tumor that
Laetrile had failed to control. Laetrile, it would seem, had
not only proved ineffective, but had proved so where many
other drugs had succeeded. Such a notion, however, is a
serious distortion of the truth.

A review of the literature published on the CD_8F_1 experimental tumor system at the time of Sloan-Kettering's press
conference reveals that the primary spontaneous tumor, treated in the same animal in which it arose, had proved extremely
resistant to the effects of many known powerful anti-cancer
agents (14). So resistant was the spontaneous tumor that it
had been "largely shelved" as a methodology of screening substances for anti-cancer activity, presumably because its
great resistance to such effects might mean that agents that
had considerable promise in cancer treatment might not reveal
that promise against the tumor.

The CD_8F_1 tumor system against which the eight agents
referred to in the original Sloan-Kettering paper had shown
effects was in fact not the spontaneous tumor treated in the
host animal, but a system in which a tumor from a mature female was transplanted to a young male and treated as soon as
a day later. These so-called "early" transplantable tumors
were described by Daniel Martin, who had pioneered in working
with the CD_8F_1 mouse strain, as "the most sensitive in pick-
ing up anti-cancer activity" (14). Thus, it appeared that the
Sloan-Kettering paper was comparing the negative results of
Laetrile in the most resistant CD_8F_1 tumor test with the
positive results of other drugs in the least resistant CD_8F_1
test, a comparison in which Laetrile would be certain to
suffer, and which would seem to make an especially strong
case for keeping Laetrile from being clinically tried.

The publication of the Second Opinion report on Laetrile and the subsequent dismissal of Ralph Moss from Sloan-Kettering's public affairs department was followed, in early December of 1977, by the publication of an article in The Sciences, the magazine of the New York Academy of Sciences, which had been conducting an independent investigation of the handling of Laetrile research at Sloan-Kettering. Although this article did not challenge the overall verdict of Sloan-Kettering on Laetrile, it did call attention to the unusual circumstances and form of the cancer center's publication of their results, and especially to the misleading paragraph about the CD_8F_1 spontaneous tumor system. The article concluded:

> Differences of interpretation are a legitimate and inevitable part of the scientific process. But when they seem to be offered in response to public or political pressure, science suffers and so, ultimately, does the public which depends on it (15, p. 13).

The Sciences' article prompted Lawrence Altman, a physician reporter at the New York Times to interview Chester Stock about the misleading statement. Stock explained that it had originated with Daniel Martin. "We accepted the statement from Dr. Martin as submitted," Stock told The Times, "I did not check the original publications to be certain of the appropriateness of the statement. It should not have been used in the context of this report, and therefore it has been deleted" (16). Stock credited the appearance of the statement to Daniel Martin's "overenthusiasm."

Herbert Kayden, a cardiologist and then president of the New York Academy of Sciences, taking care to remark that "there is nothing that warrants Laetrile as a useful agent in the treatment of cancer," characterized Martin's statement as a "procedural error" and said that the "misinterpretation by Dr. Martin was not excusable." He praised Chester Stock for his commitment to removing the misleading paragraph from the journal version of the Sloan-Kettering paper (16).

Kayden's concern was echoed in the medical press. Derek Cassels, clinical editor of The Medical Post, a fortnightly review of medical news and opinion published in Canada, wrote in a full-page editorial that "like Caesar's wife, the way a scientific argument is put must be above reproach. This is particularly true when it is being used to shoot at another thesis -- one widely thought to be false."

"We sympathize with investigators who are working under

pressure from inside and outside an institution 'to produce,'" the editorial concluded, "But it is in such a situation where there is an enormous amount of public scrutiny
that their findings must be absolutely honest" (17).

In the version of the paper published in the Journal of
Surgical Oncology, the paragraph was removed, and the following addendum explained:

   The CD_8F_1 murine spontaneous mammary cancer
is an animal tumor model with clinical therapeutic
predictive ability because the anti-cancer agents
considered clinically active against human breast
cancer also are effective against this murine
breast cancer. Therefore, in this therapeutically
relevant animal tumor model, the finding that
Laetrile is devoid of anti-cancer activity is
particularly pertinent.

   In the original pre-publication version of
this paper the paragraph making the above point
did not state that the test system, which established the unique therapeutic correlations between this animal tumor and human cancer findings,
employs first generation tumor transplants. That
paragraph placed within the context of a report on
spontaneous animal tumors was interpreted by some
to indicate that the therapeutic correlations were
determined on the murine spontaneous tumor system
per se; therefore, that paragraph has been deleted
from the paper so as not to be misleading in this
regard (13, p. 122).

The Sloan-Kettering experience with Laetrile, characterized by journalist Nicholas Wade of Science as "a painful
case of overexposure," (3, p. 1231) appears to have been one
in which the political and scientific domains inter-penetrat-
ed and affected each other's processes to a far greater
extent than usual. This view has perhaps been best expressed
by Robert Good, president and director of the Sloan-Kettering
Institute: "I sure as hell wish the Sloan-Kettering Insti-
ture had not taken on the testing," he said. "It's been such
a bag of worms. It has nothing to do with science; it has
to do with politics" (3, p. 1231).

References and Notes

1. Federal Code (1978), Title 21, Food and Drugs, part 312,
    New Drugs for Investigational Use, subpart A, exemptions
    from section 505(a), 312.1, paragraph 6a; part 314, New

Drug Applications, subpart A, general provisions, 314.1, paragraph 2.d.ii and 314.10, paragraph b.

2. Office of Cancer Communications, NCI Testing of Laetrile in Animals (National Cancer Institute, Bethesda, 1977).

3. N. Wade, "Laetrile at Sloan-Kettering: A Question of Ambiguity," Science 198, 1231-1234 (23 December 1977).

4. B. J. Culliton, "Sloan-Kettering: The Trials of an Apricot Pit - 1973," Science 182, 1000-1003 (7 December 1973).

5. E. Holles, "Birch Society Members Tied to Smuggling of Illegal Drug," New York Times (1 June 1976), p. 18.

6. The Committee for Freedom of Choice in Cancer Therapy, Anatomy of a Cover-Up: Successful Sloan-Kettering Amygdalin (Laetrile) Animal Studies (Los Altos, California, 1975).

7. F. Ingelfinger, "Laetrilomania," New England Journal of Medicine 296, 1168 (19 May 1977).

8. C. C. Stock, G. S. Tarnowski, F. A. Schmid, D. J. Hutchinson, and M. N. Teller, "Anti-tumor Tests of Amygdalin in Transplantable Animal Tumor Systems," unpublished manuscript, Sloan-Kettering Institute, 1977.

9. C. C. Stock, D. S. Martin, K. Sugiura, R. A. Fugman, I. Mountain, E. Stockert, F. A. Schmid, and G. S. Tarnowski, "Anti-tumor Tests of Amygdalin in Spontaneous Animal Tumor Systems," unpublished manuscript, Sloan-Kettering Institute, 1977.

10. Second Opinion, Second Opinion Special Report: Laetrile at Sloan-Kettering (New York, 1977).

11. Second Opinion Newsletter 2 (June, 1977).

12. See note 3 and personal communication.

13. C. C. Stock, D. S. Martin, K. Sugiura, R. A. Fugman, I. M. Mountain, E. Stockert, F. A. Schmid, and G. S. Tarnowski, "Anti-tumor Tests of Amygdalin in Spontaneous Animal Tumor Systems," Journal of Surgical Oncology 10,90 (1978).

14. D. S. Martin, P. Hayworth and R. A. Fugman, "Solid Tumor Animal Model Therapeutically Predictive for Human Breast Cancer," Cancer Chemotherapy Reports 5, 90 (December 1978).

15. R. D. Smith, "The Laetrile Papers," The Sciences 18, 10-13 (January 1978).

16. L. Altman, "Laetrile Study Data Faced by Challenge," New York Times (13 December 1977).

17. D. Cassels, "The Selling of Caesar's Wife," The Medical Post (3 January 1978), p. 1.

4. The Political Implications of Laetrile: Who Gets What, When and How

We in the Public Health Services are concerned
about the increasing use of Laetrile by cancer
patients in this country.

Laetrile is a cyanide-containing substance derived
from apricot and other fruit kernels. Its proponents say that it is effective in the prevention,
cure or control of cancer.

No evidence to support these claims has ever been
submitted to the Food and Drug Administration.
The National Cancer Institute has conducted five
tests on Laetrile and concluded that it is ineffective in animal systems. There have been many
other tests of Laetrile in animals, and FDA and
NCI have even looked at the records of patients
who have used Laetrile to see whether there is
any evidence at all that it works.

We have found none. And in fact there is considerable evidence that it does not work.

> Julius Richmond, M.D.
> *Assistant Secretary of Health*

...The problem is that one side, the side that
opposes Laetrile, is in control of the government,
and is using it to suppress the other. In no other
area is it more obvious that the government should
be kept out. Once again, your editors are not
physicians, and do not know whether Laetrile is the
answer to cancer or not. But whether or not it is
should be decided not by government force -- but by
free physicians working with their patients and in

their laboratories. Why is it that the U.S.
Supreme Court says physicians may perform abortions,
on the ground that the physician-patient relationship is inviolable -- but that the same physician
is not permitted to prescribe Laetrile for his
patients...not to destroy life but to save it? Why
are we told that a patient has the 'right to die
with dignity,' but may not take Laetrile in an
attempt to live? Indeed, also because of government
intervention and suppression, smugglers are now selling Laetrile which therapists have found defective.

Let's return medicine to the doctors, and patients,
before cancer victims and their relatives begin hang-
ing F.D.A. medicrats from trees.

Alan Stang
American Opinion
(Conservative Journal of Public Affairs)

The quotes cited above help to summarize the highly
charged and often emotional debate over the legalization of
Laetrile in the U.S. over the last three years. This debate
has been most intensive at the State level. Forty-one states
have acted on legislative proposals to legalize the sale of
Laetrile in their particular states. As of March 1979, 22
states had rejected such proposals for legalization, and by
the summer, 21 states had acted positively on them.

How does one explain the "success" of the Laetrile proponents in their efforts to legalize Laetrile at the State
level? Is it a case of challenging the power of "big government" represented by the United States Food and Drug Administration (FDA)? Is it part of a nation-wide movement toward
deregulation? Is it part of a more global strategy to challenge the mandate of the FDA: to insure that all drugs meet
the criteria of being safe and efficacious? This paper will
address these questions from the perspective of each of the
major actors in the "Laetrile controversy."

It is very clear that the issue of whether to legalize
Laetrile and, more importantly, the questions that are being
raised in the context of debating this issue, can best be
understood when thought of as a classical political controversy (1). There are competing claims for resolution of an
issue which is "of great importance" to several different
groups, each of which is recognized to have a "legitimate
position." None of the positions can be considered to be a
priori "right" or "wrong." Political actors (decision-makers)
face the dilemma of having the formal/legal responsibility of

reconciling these competing "legitimate positions." Thus,
the process of reaching a decision (i.e., a compromise or
the decision to adopt one of the competing claims) is as
important as the substance of the decision that is ultimately
taken.

In the case of Laetrile, there is an important additional political dimension. From the perspective of the federal
government and some state governments, the Laetrile movement
can be characterized as a political disease: Laetrile is,
therefore, only a symptom of a larger political disease,
which can be described in terms similar to those used to
characterize cancer: it is dreaded, its roots stem from
many areas (dissatisfaction with government, the medical profession, and "scientific testing procedures"), and it evokes
a great deal of emotion and misunderstanding. Most importantly, this "political disease" is not open to a single cure
and certainly not the traditional ones (i.e., more regulation) that have been employed in the past.

This paper is devoted to exploring the politics behind
the Laetrile movement: what is at stake, and for whom? Who
are the major actors and what assumptions are they making
about the nature of Laetrile and the "Laetrile movement"?
In what arena is the Laetrile issue being debated, and why
was this arena chosen? What can be expected in the future?

Model of Analysis

One can learn a great deal about politics and the political implications of an issue by analyzing the definition
of the problem put forward by each of the major actors who
have a stake in the ultimate outcome of a particular decision. Problem definitions are based on assumptions about
the "causes" of a problem and where they lie. Studies have
shown that the way a problem is defined determines the
attempts at remediation, suggesting both the foci and the
techniques of intervention and by ruling out alternative
possibilities (2). More specifically, problem definitions
determine the strategy that is adopted to bring about change
in a particular issue area (3). It would also seem to follow
that whoever can have his/her definition of the problem
accepted as the basis of decision-making will have the most
to gain when a decision is taken. However, it may also be
the case that "integrative modes" of problem solving are
employed so as to emphasize collaborative solutions -- how
opposing parties can both gain -- as opposed to distributive
solutions where only one gains at the expense of another (4).

Much of this paper will be devoted to illustrating how

the Laetrile controversy can be viewed in terms of a set of conflicting problem definitions by several key actors (groups).

Before exploring the conflicting assumptions inherent in this movement, it is worth describing the background of this controversy and the areas over which there are no disagreements.

Political Background/History

The terms Laetrile and amygdalin are often used interchangeably (5). Ernst T. Krebs, Sr., a California physician, first attempted to use Laetrile as a cancer treatment in 1920. However, the drug, as extracted from apricot pits, was too toxic for human use. Dr. Krebs' son, Ernst T. Krebs, Jr., developed a purified form of Laetrile which was less toxic and advocated it as an effective treatment for cancer.

In 1961, Mr. Krebs, Jr., doing business with his father as the John Beard Memorial Foundation, and the Foundation, were both convicted of illegally promoting another drug -- "Vitamin B-15" -- for improving the performance of race horses. The U.S. District Court of San Francisco fined Mr. Krebs, Jr., and the Foundation $3,750 and put Mr. Krebs on probation for three years. As a condition of probation he was prohibited from shipping any new drugs, including Laetrile, without first having it approved by the FDA (6).

In April 1970, the McNaughton Foundation of Montreal, Canada, and Sausalito, California, claimed an exemption to sponsor a clinical trial of amygdalin (7). FDA reviewed the claim (IND) and promptly denied it because of inadequate safety testing and other deficiencies.

Yet within six years after the IND was denied, Alaska legalized the use of Laetrile. By March 1979 a total of 19 states had legalized the drug and there had been amendments or bills introduced in at least 41 states.

Competing Sets of Problem Definitions

Given the political history involved with legalizing Laetrile, one is interested in how the Laetrile "issue" has been defined by the major actors involved with it: the FDA, the proponents of legalization, state legislatures, public interest groups, and medical experts. Each of the problem definitions reflects central assumptions about the nature of the problem and the actions that need to be taken to effectively deal with it. Some of the definitions are complemen-

tary (a collaborative solution), and some are clearly distributive (a competitive solution).

Definition I. Laetrile as a Scientific Controversy

One perspective on the Laetrile issue is that this is
purely a scientific matter and should be dealt with on scientific grounds. One needs to go through regular drug testing procedures (i.e., NDA, IND) and determine the safety and
efficacy of Laetrile.

This view of the issue would lead one to concentrate
almost exclusively on the scientific and technical aspects
of Laetrile. Is it efficacious? Is it safe? If so, under
what conditions? What types of animal and/or human tests
should be sanctioned to prove the efficacy and safety of
Laetrile? Should a retrospective study of medical records
be undertaken to test the safety of this issue?

It is clear that on the formal level, the FDA must
appear to be accepting this definition of the problem. The
FDA is specifically prohibited by law against lobbying in
state legislative actions. It is also prohibited from lobbying in the U.S. Congress. However, on the informal level,
the FDA surely could encourage its supporters within HEW and
the Congress to take the more general political implications
of this issue quite seriously.

However, we have found no evidence of a broader view of
the problem -- even at the highest levels of the FDA. A
relatively recent internal memorandum from the Commissioner
of Food and Drugs to the Secretary of HEW starts off by concentrating on these scientific aspects:

> As you know, Laetrile is a compound known as
> amygdalin, a glycoside that can readily be
> extracted from apricot pits and some other
> natural sources. It can be manufactured on
> virtually cottage industry basis, and "standards"
> for its production undoubtedly vary widely; that
> is one reason why it is difficult to persuade
> believers that a given test has really proven its
> lack of efficacy. Five animal studies done at NCI
> on Laetrile have shown no anti-tumor activity.
> Now NCI is quietly arranging a well-controlled
> human study, for which we are in the process of
> granting an IND. About three INDs for this com-
> pound have been received by FDA since 1963, none
> of them with any convincing efficacy evidence (8).

This memo was summary document of the FDA's views and recommendations to the Secretary of Health, Education, and Welfare. As cited in this essay, similar presentations of the problem were made in a public announcement by the Assistant Secretary of Health.

Action Implications

The action implications which follow from this definition of the problem are fairly straight-forward and clear:

- Sanction and conduct all medical tests/ experiments which seem warranted within the boundaries of the Food, Drug, and Cosmetic Act of 1962. The FDA has done this and even gone beyond it in helping NCI plan for a retrospective case review. FDA officials would contend that this represents their political concession, because of the high emotional content of the issue.

- Conduct a public education campaign on the dangers of Laetrile. The FDA has undertaken a massive educational campaign to warn the public against the dangers of taking Laetrile. As part of this effort, a poster was produced to warn people about Laetrile.

- Testify in front of state legislatures in which they are invited to testify. Since 1976, the FDA has made approximately 50 presentations of facts, figures, and perspectives in various state legislatures. These presentations reflect the FDA definition of the problem. They recognize the political issues, but deal with them by trying to concentrate on the scientific evidence. For example, on the highly volatile issue of freedom of choice, FDA officials would give the following testimony:

   The issue of 'freedom of choice' is not a valid one as it relates to Laetrile. The concept of freedom is being debased by swindling those who are desperate for their lives. The choice should be among products recognized to be effective. For the believing but uninformed cancer victim, he may be choosing death with Laetrile versus

the possibility of life with other cancer
treatment methods known to be more effective.

Again, the FDA is concentrating on efficacy even when trying
to discuss the political implications of the issue (8).

● Conducting research and making educational materials
available to the public and any legislator on
request.

Definition II. Laetrile as a Quack Cure

A second perspective on the problem, held by a smaller
number of FDA officials and some legislators is that Laetrile is just another in a series of quack cures.

In its 70-year history, the FDA has put hundreds of
"cures" out of business. It appears that (from the perspective of FDA officials and others who define the problem in
this fashion) approximately every ten years, one "cure,"
usually for cancer, is promoted so effectively that it becomes a national issue. The most recent, prior to Laetrile,
was Krebiozen, and prior to that, the "Hoxsey Treatment" and
the "Koch Treatment." It is interesting to note that, similar to Laetrile, the Hoxsey treatments continued to be
offered by practitioners in Mexico even after the sale of
the material was judged illegal in the United States.

Those who define the Laetrile issue in this fashion
continue to concentrate on the scientific evidence; by concentrating on "quackery" they feel they are taking the political aspects of the issue into account. The quackery issue
is the one "political hazard" cited by the Commissioner in
his memo to the Secretary of HEW:

If one says that Laetrile can escape the efficacy
requirement, one opens the door for every quack
cure imaginable. In Nevada, Gerovital H even got
piggy-backed onto the Laetrile legislation while
it was being drafted; I can see no logical place
to draw the line short of repealing the Kefauver-
Harris amendments (8).

Quackery is also of some concern because some FDA officials believe that the agency could have "nipped [Laetrile]
in the bud" many years ago by "taking prompt actions against
Laetrile's early promoters." When asked why this wasn't
done, one official replied that "it was viewed as an insig-
nificant problem ... we had bigger fish to fry in other
areas, such as in drug compliance actions and food safety."

Another FDA official said that quackery was given a relatively low priority at that time. He said, "This was a delib-
erate decision because of limitations of manpower. In terms
of benefit/risk, the emphasis was put on drugs" (9).

Action Implications

Most of the action implications which follow from this
definition of the problem are an extension of the ones
based on the "scientific perspective":

- Include this element in the public education
  campaigns and in testimony before the state
  legislatures. The FDA has done this fairly
  consistently. It tries to inform the public
  and their elected representatives of the
  similarities between Laetrile and other so-
  called quack cures.

- Convince the Secretary of HEW and the Assistant Secretary of Health of the importance
  of this problem. The FDA has certainly done
  this.

- Increase the resources devoted to combating
  the "Laetrile movement." In the short-turn
  the FDA has devoted substantial resources to
  public education, testimony before state
  legislatures, and legal as well as compliance
  actions.

- Consider devoting more resources to combating
  "quackery" in the future. This is a long-term
  proposal and is being given serious consideration within the FDA.

Definition III. Freedom of Choice

There is a group of proponents for the legalization of
Laetrile who concentrate on what they call "the freedom of
choice" issue. "Freedom of choice" has several different
meanings: (a) the right of a doctor to prescribe whatever
treatment that he/she deems to be effective for a particular
patient; (b) the freedom of a patient to choose whichever
doctor and, by implication, treatment that he chooses--
the government should not interfere in this choice; and (c)
at a maximum, government intervention should only involve
providing the public with information--"on all sides of the
question," and the public should then be able to make an
informed choice.

Organizations have been formed to represent this point of view. These organizations are growing in size and number. At this writing, the Committee for Freedom of Choice in Cancer Therapy claims to have 450 chapters and 23,000 members and is one of the main actors in the effort to legalize Laetrile. Other groups have also been formed to join in their common goal to legalize Laetrile. Several of the largest are the International Association of Cancer Victims and Friends, the Cancer Control Society, and the National Health Federation.

These groups, which have tens of thousands of members or supporters, publish periodic journals; hold social and business meetings, conventions, etc; and apply pressure on cancer patients and their families, in some instances within 24 hours after diagnosis, to use Laetrile.

Several points should be made about those who define the problem in this fashion:

1. Laetrile is basically a convenient vehicle to help reach a larger, and broader set of ends. The freedom of choice issues are at stake and not Laetrile qua Laetrile.

2. This group does not make any particular claims for the efficacy of Laetrile. Instead, they concentrate on alternative treatments to conventional cancer therapy. They offer a whole package of treatments including diet, and nutritional packages. It is almost as if they are trying to form a culture around the non-traditional treatment of cancer (10).

3. They are challenging long-standing government policies and methods of regulation.

4. This point of view enjoys a good deal of public support. The New York Times and the Detroit Free Press have come out editorially in favor of Laetrile and the Harris Poll reflects substantial support from the public at large. In addition, a survey taken by Cambridge Reports, Inc., asked the following question: "Some people say companies should tell us in plain English what the possible dangers are in a product, as they do on cigarette packages, and then leave it to us as individuals to decide whether or not we want to use that product. Would you agree or disagree?" Eighty-two percent of the respondents

agreed, 9 percent said they didn't know, and 9
percent disagreed.

Action Implications

This group of advocates is extremely careful in the tactics it employs and can also be characterized as being very
shrewd political analysts. Their definition of the problem
has led them to adopt the following action strategies:

1. Organize letter-writing campaigns to legis-
    lators in the states where Laetrile legis-
    lation is being considered.

2. Organize testimony before the state legis-
    latures -- both testimonials by those who
    have used Laetrile and testimony on the
    issue of freedom of choice.

3. Organize and recruit members at the grass-
    roots level. This involves contacting
    recently diagnosed cancer patients and
    encouraging to accept non-traditional forms
    of therapy and encouraging to join the
    "appropriate organization."

4. Working at the national level to insure
    that "freedom of choice" may become a
    reality. At a United States Senate hearing
    on July 12, 1977, this group's position was
    presented by Robert W. Bradford, President
    of the Committee for Freedom of Choice in
    Cancer Therapy, Inc.:

    "The FDA MUST get off the backs of physi-
    cians, cancer patients, and ourselves.
    What, in the name of humanity, is this
    agency doing? Whom does it represent?
    Surely, not the people. The Harris Poll
    has already indicated that. How is it
    possible that at a time when our nation
    is flooded with heroin, cocaine, uppers
    and downers and is literally awash in
    marijuana, the federal government sees
    fit to expend millions and millions of
    dollars of taxpayer funds to suppress
    the extract of apricot kernels? Where
    is the logic? Where is the morality?" (11).

5. Working at the national level for legislation which
    might help insure for freedom of choice. The

group is advocating amendments to the New
Drug bill currently being considered by
Congress. This group would like the efficacy clause of the Food and Drug act to be
omitted.

Definition IV. Big Government Interference

The last definition of the Laetrile issue which has been
prevalent over the last number of years is the one which
stipulates that big government interferes far too much and
often in "our lives." Laetrile is simply an example of a
more general trend toward government interference in our
lives.

The groups representing this point of view are many of
the same that were listed above. In addition, this broader
definition of the problem allows the advocates of deregulation to become "part of the coalition." While some people
in journalistic and academic spheres may not fully accept
the definition of the problem in terms of freedom of choice,
they are sympathetic to deregulation.

Action Implications

In addition to all of the tactics listed above, this
group would work toward broad-scale public support through
educational campaigns and generalized legislation. Examples
of their success include political erosion of the efficacy
and safety provisions of the Food, Drug, and Cosmetic Act:
(1) the 1974 vitamin amendments which limits the authority
of the FDA to classify a vitamin as a drug solely because it
exceeds the level of potency which the Secretary (HEW) determines is nutritionally rational or useful; (2) the
saccharin 18-month moratorium passed by Congress. The
Delaney Clause of the F, D & C Act prohibits the use of any
food additive (i.e., saccharin) which is known to produce
cancer (regardless of dose) in man or animals. There have
been several animal experiments in which cancer has been
produced in animals by high doses of saccharin. Because of
a public groundswell against the immediate implementation
of a saccharin ban as a food additive and to allow further
testing, Congress passed the 18-month moratorium.

It is possible that further challenges such as from
Laetrile could lead to the abolishment or modification of
the current efficacy requirements for new drugs. In fact, a
proposal has been introduced in the House of Representatives
with 100 cosigners which would abolish the efficacy provision
requirement for new drugs. Such a bill, if enacted, would,

according to FDA officials, negate much of the agency efforts
to provide effective drugs to the American public and even
lead to a) the resumption of "quack" medical drugs distributed in interstate commerce, or b) exemptions granted for
specific items; i.e., Laetrile.

The Debate Over Laetrile

The debate over Laetrile is occuring at several levels
utilizing several different definitions of the problem: (1)
at the state level the FDA-supplied definitions (I, II) are
in direct conflict with the definitions of the proponents
of legalizing Laetrile (III, IV); and (2) at the federal
level more general legislation is being considered; clearly,
the proponents are "having their day in court" for the broader definitions of the problem.

In examining these legislative debates, we analyzed the
legislation in each state which has considered a bill to
legalize Laetrile (e.g., what provisions were included, which
provisions were deleted during debate). Moreover, in three
states, face-to-face interviews were conducted with all principal actors: legislators, the governor's office, officials
from the State Department of Health, Bureau of Drugs, and
pressure/lobby groups. Face-to-face interviews were also
conducted at the federal level with representatives from each
FDA division involved with this controversy. The FDA moni-
tored the Laetrile debates in each state considering such
legislation. Consequently, we were also able to collect FDA
data on all of the states debating Laetrile legislation:
which actors were involved, what positions were taken, and
what implementation procedures were adopted.

The State Level

The Legislation

The debate over the legalization of the sale of Laetrile
has followed a rather typical pattern in the states that have
considered it. The bill is usually introduced by a Senator
or Representative who personally has cancer or who has a
relative who has been diagnosed as having cancer.

The proposed legislation typically calls for: (1) protecting physicians; (2) protecting pharmacists; (3) requiring
a prescription; (4) permitting its manufacturing within a
state; (5) making provisions for quality control; (6) desig-
nating an agency responsible for monitoring and implementation; (7) requiring written informed consent or records; (8)

requiring that containers of Laetrile be labelled with the statement: "Amygdalin has not been approved as a treatment or cure of any malignancy, disease, illness, or physical condition by the United States Food and Drug Administration."

Federal statutes prohibit states from importing Laetrile (an exception to this is the recent order by Judge Bohannan which stipulates that Laetrile may be imported for use on terminally ill cancer patients). Therefore, in order not to be in violation of federal law, Laetrile sold "in-state" must be completely manufactured within the state itself.

The Role of the FDA

Once a bill has been introduced, the FDA has proceeded to make its position very clear. Although the FDA cannot actively lobby in a state legislative action, it will, if asked, provide technical assistance or testify at hearings. The FDA can also, upon request, assist state legislative committees by providing factual information.

The FDA has provided such assistance in almost every state considering Laetrile legislation. The interviews conducted at the state level reveal that because the agency believes that Laetrile is a most dangerous type of health fraud, it has expanded technical assistance resources to states in order to prevent or postpone passage of, or to weaken, Laetrile bills.

In fact, the FDA has done everything in its power to indicate how strongly it feels--ranging from technical assistance, to testimony, to telegrams to Governors, and in making it very clear what its legal options were. A telegram from Commissioner Kennedy to Governor Du Pont of Delaware is typical:

> Should Delaware legalize Laetrile, a great
> number of cancer victims in the state could be
> irreparably harmed, both by spending large sums
> of money for this drug and foregoing known
> effective treatments that are now available for
> many forms of cancer, especially in early stages.
> I hope that Delaware would not legitimize this
> exploitation of a tragic disease. Its [Laetrile]
> shipment from or into Delaware is now illegal
> under federal law and passage of state legisla-
> tion would not alter this situation (8).

With this telegram, the Commissioner of the FDA stated explicitly that his agency was strongly opposed to promoting

Laetrile; more importantly, perhaps, he reminded the states
what the limits and powers of the federal law were.

Our interviews reveal that, in informal conversations,
some FDA officials would consider regulatory action to control local efforts to manufacture Laetrile if evidence of
federal jurisdiction over any of the drug's components could
be found. If inert ingredients, containers, or labels used
for the production of the product were from interstate sources,
they were prepared to consider obtaining injunctions to halt
manufacturing operations.

The role of the FDA is complicated. It is not merely
acting as would a scientist in a technical discussion. It is
acting on the basis of enabling legislation passed by the
U.S. Congress. There is not much inclination in Congress to
change this legislation. The FDA is acting as a political
actor as well as a scientific/technical actor.

In this respect the FDA's role should be differentiated
from that of a State Department of Health and/or Bureau of
Drugs. The State Bureaus have not been acting under any enabling legislation. Indeed, they have acted in what might be
considered "direct contradiction" of a legislative act. In
the case of the States, the legislature is the political actor
and the State Bureau of Drugs represents the scientific or
technical actor.

Other Testimony

In most states, the legislature has been quite thorough
in investigating the controversy. Testimony is sought from
all concerned parties. Thus, state medical associations, consumer groups, Deans of Medical Schools, and individual citizens treated with Laetrile are heard from. The testimony
taken ranges from complex scientific evidence, to expert opinion by Deans, to testimonials by cancer victims.

The Role of Government

Governors of states took on very different roles in this
controversy. Some did not want to get involved with the controversy and simply followed the lead of the legislature;
these governors usually signed the bills into law without
comment. Others vetoed the legislation reemphasizing many
of the same messages highlighted by the FDA. Governor James
Thompson of Illinois was typical of this group of Governors:

> ....Lastly, if Laetrile is legalized in spite of
> all scientific evidence to the contrary, then
> what logic stands in the way of legalizing any

supposed cancer treatment which can marshall
sufficient personal testimony and the necessary
advertising dollars. Why not permit the sale of
sawdust or Vitamin A as cures for cancer...on
the ground that the terminally ill should be permitted freedom of choice (8).

Legalizing the Sale of Laetrile - The Implementation Phase

As already indicated, each bill designated an agency
responsible for implementing the law passed by the legislature. Usually this was the State Department of Health.

Some states did not adopt any specific regulations or
rules to govern the implementation of the Laetrile legislation. These states relied on existing state regulations or
they simply adopted the FDA safety and efficacy standards.
The FDA regulations were often adopted on the premise that
they were proven and should be adopted at the state level.

However, in three states, the Director of the Bureau of
Drugs, acting for the Commissioner of Health, adopted specific regulations to guide the implementation of the Laetrile
legislation. The three states vary only slightly in their
behavior at this stage of development:

State I

The State Health Department has delegated to their
Bureau of Drugs the responsibility for implementing and enforcing the Laetrile Act. The state official who is Director of the Bureau of Drugs is a nationally recognized
scientist and administrator. He has published many professional articles concerning drugs, and has recently been
elected president of a multi-state Health Association.

The Director, on the basis of the available scientific
evidence, emphatically believes that "Laetrile is not only
worthless in the treatment of cancer, but that it is a health
fraud; and worse still, citizens in the state are foregoing
conventional treatment in favor of Laetrile with fatal results."

The Laetrile Act did not change any existing drug laws
in the state. The old state drug law does have a safety requirement for "new drugs" produced in intra-state commerce.
However, this part of the law has not been enforced in over
twenty years because the FDA safety regulations were applied
in the state. These FDA regulations require an extensive
work-up on the toxicity and toxicology of all new drugs
prior to distribution in inter-state commerce. The limits

of exclusive intra-state use of a drug is illustrated by the
Director's comment that "he can only remember during the past
twenty years, only two requests for state approval of a new
drug...and in both cases he convinced the applicant not to
apply." However, two applications have been received by the
Division of Drugs for approval to manufacture Laetrile in the
state. Both companies have followed up their initial requests with phone calls and letters.

Prior to any response to the two manufacturers, the
state Director, Bureau of Drugs, has, with the concurrence
of the Health Commissioner, promulgated, without public
hearings, regulations under the existing "old" state drug
laws pertaining to the safety of intra-state new drugs. "In
effect," the Director said, "even if a company were able to
do this (i.e., meet the safety tests), the approval and legal
use of Laetrile in the state could be delayed from three to
eleven years." The FDA experience is that it takes an aver-
age of seven to eight years for a 'new drug' to be approved.

Our interviews with State and Federal (FDA) officials
reveal the following critical facts:
1.   This Director of Drugs is a nationally known scientist and, hence, any actions he takes may be followed by
other officials (bureaucrats) in states that have Laetrile
Acts.
2.   There is no question that the Director of the State
Bureau of Drugs has consciously contradicted legislative
intent. He is neither embarrassed nor secretive about the
fact that these new regulations were adopted specifically to
stop the widespread usage of Laetrile.
3.   In effect, he has taken actions "so that the state
will have time to realize that Laetrile is a most dangerous
hoax and health fraud and will repeal the law." His actions
are based on the commitment to lives which will be saved by
conventional cancer treatments rather than lost because of
Laetrile.

State II

The situation in another state that we examined was
almost exactly the same as the one just described (including
a nationally recognized scientist being involved) except for
the fact that the Governor had vetoed the bill and the legislature overrode the veto.

State III

In the third state that we looked into, the top state
officials adopted a somewhat different tactic in response to
the passing of the Laetrile Act. The Director, under the

quality control authority of the Laetrile Act, with the concurrence of the Health Commission and without public hearings, adopted by reference the Good Manufacturing Practices regulations of the FDA. These regulations require that Laetrile manufacturers have <u>adequately</u> equipped facilities, <u>adequately</u> trained technical and professional personnel, the <u>necessary</u> analytical controls and <u>adequate</u> record keeping methods. Laetrile not manufactured under conforming methods or in conforming facilities is considered adulterated and will be seized and destroyed by the state. Our interviews indicate that these regulations were adopted with the explicit intent of delaying the distribution of Laetrile in the state.

In effect. Laetrile is not available in the United States except for patients who have a doctor's affidavit that they are terminally ill. Laetrile is available in Mexico and Europe. Cancer victims not classified as terminally ill by a physician have to rely upon these supplies.

Clearly, this type of scenario just described is not necessarily typical for each state that legalizes the sale of Laetrile.

The Legislative Response

For purposes of implementation there are two possible ways to interpret legislation legalizing Laetrile: (1) "The legislative intent" was to make the drug Laetrile immediately available for public use; (2) The legislative intent was to make the drug available only after it had been tested for <u>safety</u>.

In the three states included in this study, the public officials responsible for implementation <u>all</u> interpreted legislative intent as requiring "vigorous scientific testing" for safety. From their perspective, this should be required despite the delay it would cause in making Laetrile available for use by the general public.

The officials formulated these regulations knowing that the legislators might not understand the full implications of them for "delays" in marketing the drug. One official from a State Bureau of Drugs reported:

> The legislature is aware of the new regulations but, as of yet, is not cognizant of the FDA experience in terms of granting "new drug" approval (average 7-8 years) or the state intention to 'literally' enforce Good Manufacturing practices

on Laetrile manufacturers if and whenever necessary.

It should be understood that these officials promulgated
the regulations with the specific intent of blocking the
widespread use of Laetrile. These actions were taken on the
basis of a commitment and belief that Laetrile represented a
"hoax" and a "dangerous health fraud."

Given this background, the state legislators who were
the primary sponsors of the legislation to legalize Laetrile
were re-interviewed. The interviewer inquired: "Since the
passage of legislation to legalize the sale of Laetrile in
your state, what has been done to implement this law? What
role have you played in the implementation process?"

These interviews with the prime sponsors in three states
revealed:
(1) All of the legislators were aware of the activities
of the State Department of Health;
(2) They were all aware of the details of the regulations and the fact that the public distribution of Laetrile
would be delayed by seven to eight years; and
(3) They were all familiar with the scientific evidence
presented by the FDA, the AMA, and local medical professionals. On the basis of this evidence, most of them believed
that Laetrile was not efficacious and that the FDA testing
was "valid."

However, despite the fact that they were all strong
supporters of the initial legislation, they were not going
to challenge the regulations promulgated by the officials
from the Department of Health through any of the means available to them.

In this context, it is worth noting that legislators
were not defenseless against the actions of the state bureaucrats. They could hold public hearings on the regulations,
force the bureaucrats to reformulate the proposed regulations, they could "go to the press," or they could encourage
supporters to challenge these regulations in court. The
legislators interviewed knew of their options and consciously
chose not to act on them. One respondent seemed to characterize the general attitude of the strong legislative supporters of legalizing Laetrile: "I have done my job; others
now have to address the problem."

The Federal Level

At the federal level, the FDA has been very active;
however, there has been no specific legislation concerning

the legalization of Laetrile. Instead, as already discussed
Congress is considering a new drug law and there are propo-
sals to repeal the efficacy clause of the Food, Drug, and
Cosmetic Act.

The FDA fears that people have lost sight of the history
behind the Food, Drug, and Cosmetic Act. The 1962 Drug Amendments were enacted following the Thalidomide disaster. The use
of Thalidomide, a sedative, by pregnant women causes severe de-
formity of the child. Although the drug was never approved for
interstate commercial use, it was then legal to distribute the
drug to physicians for experimental purposes. It was estimated
that the drug was given to over 3800 U.S. women of child-
bearing age, nine of whom gave birth to malformed children.
Thalidomide was approved by many other countries, with birth
deformities resulting throughout the world.

The 1962 Drug Amendments extended, expanded and strengthened the regulatory authority of the FDA. Among other
provisions, the FDA was authorized to approve a new drug
for marketing only after the sponsor had met the statuatory
requirements for safety and efficacy. Approval was condi-
tional upon the showing of "substantial evidence" of efficacy, and the burden of proof rested with the manufacturer.

The efficacy and safety provisions of the current law
are, in the opinion of the FDA, absolutely essential in
carrying out its mission of public health and safety.

There is evidence of real public concern that terminal
patients should be allowed any drug, regardless of questions
concerning its efficacy or other effects. For example, this
concept has resulted in a bill, introduced in New York State,
which would authorize physicians to administer controlled
substances such as marijuana, heroin and others to terminally
ill patients. The current practice of careful allocation of
"pain killers" for terminally ill patients is, according to
Alan G. Hevesi, Chairman of the New York Assembly Health Committee, "silly" because it denies "terminally ill patients
certain drugs because of the potential for addiction."

A similar argument has been made for Laetrile in that,
even though there is no scientific evidence that the drug is
useful in the treatment of cancer, proponents ask, "Why deny
the terminal patient or his/her relatives the 'straw' which
they so desperately desire?" Moreover, Laetrile very probably
produces a real placebo effect, although this effect has not
been objectively demonstrated. Oncologists and psychiatrists
have argued that Laetrile cannot be considered a safe placebo
since it drives patients away from good medical care.

A possible argument against a terminal classification of
any patient is that the subjective medical opinion of one
physician may be incorrect. The uncertainty of individual
medical opinion has also been seen in recent court cases which
attempt to ascertain if a patient is dead, so that heroic
life-support systems may be legally disconnected.

It is important to underscore the fact that the debate at
the federal level is concerned with the broader medical policy
issues. There is little concern for Laetrile qua Laetrile.
Larger and broader political ends are at stake.

The Current Legal Status of Laetrile

As the discussion of the state case histories illustrate, despite the so-called legalization of Laetrile in 22
states, Laetrile is not available on the market except for
the terminally ill.

Legal Issues

Even in those states which have legalized the manufacture of Laetrile, no Laetrile is being manufactured. The
fact that a state enacts legislation which permits the use
of Laetrile within its boundaries has no effect on the established policies of the FDA. The shipment of Laetrile from
or into a state is now illegal under federal law and passage
of state legislation does not alter this situation. Passage
of such legislation does not protect sponsors, promoters,
distributors, dispensors, or sellers of Laetrile from applicable civil or criminal sanctions under the Federal Food,
Drug, and Cosmetic Act.

The FDA is continuing to initiate legal action against
individuals and firms who are manufacturing and shipping
Laetrile illegally in interstate commerce. The largest enforcement action to date occurred on May 16, 1977, when U.S.
Marshals in Wisconsin seized approximately 12 tons of apricot
kernels, 100,000 unfilled drug capsules and several containers of partially pressed apricot kernels. On August 4, 1977,
Judge John W. Reynolds, District Judge for the Eastern District of Wisconsin, issued an injunction against numerous
defendants involved in the allegedly illegal operation. The
injunction was upheld by the 7th Circuit Court of Appeals in
December, 1977. In upholding Judge Reynolds' decision, the
7th Circuit Court considered the decision of Judge Luther Bohannon, but concluded that the public health would be endan-
gered if defendants in the Wisconsin case were permitted to
resume the manufacture and sale of Laetrile.

Political Issues

The legal status of Laetrile only represents one dimension of the problem. The other major dimension has been
acted out on the state level. Proponents have won a symbolic
victory in bringing the issue to the consciousness of the
public at large. Since Laetrile is currently not available
in any state (except for terminal patients), perhaps, given
their definitions of the problem, this symbolic victory is all
the proponents were aiming for.

However, the issues of freedom of choice and limiting big
government intervention are more generalizable, and these are
being considered at the federal level. This interpretation
would be consistent with the proponents' definition of the
problem and the implementation history at the state level.

It is true that the specific Laetrile controversy at
the state level is "dying out." However, other product-
specific legislation has been introduced in 29 states over
the last year. There has been some early research into the
use of tetrahydrocannabinol -- a marijuana based drug -- for
the treatment of after-affects of conventional cancer therapy. The FDA is considering whether to allow human testing
on this drug. States are now passing laws to legalize the
manufacturing and use of the drug before the FDA has finished its review. Four states have passed the legislation and
25 others are considering it this year.

Discussion/Conclusions

The analysis of the Laetrile movement serves to illustrate how competing definitions of a complex problem influence
policy making. In addition, it serves to guide us in our
understanding of the debate that is likely to ensue on this
and related issues in the future.

What Was at Stake?

From the point of view of the FDA, scientific standards
of safety and efficacy were at stake. Clearly, these standards were defended -- from a very narrow perspective. No
one challenged the scientific evidence concerning Laetrile
qua Laetrile.

The proponents simply make the point that there are alternative forms of therapy and there are packages of "cures"
that include Laetrile. No individual claims for Laetrile
were made.

But, the proponents were really not arguing about Laetrile. They were arguing about freedom of choice and big
government interference.

It is clear that they were able to make their definition
of the problem stick -- it is one that was accepted by the
public at large. This fact accounts for the ground swell
(i.e., grass-roots support) supporting the legalization of
Laetrile.

The State legislator, however, faced a dilemma: was he
or she to vote with the scientific evidence or with the public
pressure that was being exerted? The fact that Federal laws
apply at the state level (except for intra-state commerce)
and that state bureaucrats were in some cases not willing to
implement the Laetrile legislation helped some of the legislators out of the dilemma. They could vote for Laetrile
knowing that it would still not be available on the market
place at large.

This reality does not appear to particularly concern the
proponents of Laetrile because they too have succeeded: (1)
freedom of choice is on the minds of a great many people;
and (2) the Congress is giving serious consideration to
legislation which would serve their needs and "cause."

Which Problem Definition Prevailed?

Overall, it seems fairly clear that the proponents of
Laetrile had their definition of the problem accepted. In
the future, the FDA will have to learn to work with the
political definition of the problem if it is to defend its
broader interests and needs.

Accountability and Responsibility

The Laetrile case is most interesting for what it suggests more generally about accountability and responsibility
in public administration.

Two forms of accountability appear to be operating for
these types of issues: (a) short-term responsiveness to the
pressures and demands of the public; and (b) paternalistic
concern (long-term) for defending the interests that the
State Director of Drugs wants to protect: the ultimate health
of the public at large. As Friedrich (12) suggests, the experts need to be in a position to decide on issues that require expertise.

Although this standard of accountability is exercised
by bureaucrats (and some Governors) and accepted by legislators, the public often believes that bureaucrats are acting
autonomously and "abusing their power."

The Laetrile case suggests that our thinking about responsibility and accountability needs to be reexamined. One
perspective (13) contends that the public interest is defended through the legislative mandates of their elected
representatives. This study suggests that the public interest is defended through the actions of elected representatives in the policy making (legislative mandates) or implementation phases (formulation of regulations) of the problem
solving process; as long as the elected representatives consider the actions to be "legitimate," then the public
interest is being defended. This reformulation assumes that
the legislators are aware of what their options are during
the implementation phase, and what implications follow from
action or inaction. If elected officials are willing to
accept the professional judgment of experts, then in Finer's
terms, they are acting responsibly (13).

This case also suggests that traditional assumptions
concerning the legitimacy of paternalism need to be reexamined. The Laetrile proponents are most concerned about
the interference of big government in the lives of citizens.
Yet, the very legislators willing to pass the Laetrile Act
were also willing to allow public officials (i.e., government) to take actions that insure for the continued removal
of Laetrile from the market.

"Passing the Buck"

This apparent lack of differentiation between political
and technical responsibility is not limited to the Laetrile
issue. Other public policy issues involving scientific and
technical judgments have been handled similarly by elected
representatives -- i.e., lip-service to a position of advo-
cacy while fully expecting (or at least willing to accept)
that other political actors (e.g., the Governor, President,
a high-level bureaucrat or the courts) will take "appropriate
actions" reversing their position. Examples of this phenom-
ena include: (a) the environmental and energy issues related to granting U.S. landing rights to the Anglo-French
Concorde -- this case ended in the Courts; politicians did
not want to be on record as granting permanent landing
rights to a plane which produces noise pollution and is
energy inefficient; and (b) the siting of nuclear facilities
which are also being decided in the courts.

In the future, one should expect other issues to put politicians in the same position -- including other food and drug related issues such as vitamins, nitrites, cyclamates, etc. The politicians are sympathetic to the proponents of reducing the influence of "big government," they are willing to give lip-service to these issues. However, at the point of translating speeches into concrete programs, they recognize that the exercise of technical responsibility is the most legitimate form of public administration.

References and Notes

The author wishes to acknowledge the invaluable assistance of Robert Frankel, Deputy Associate Director of the Bureau of New Drugs, United States Food and Drug Administration, Paul Sage, FDA, and Alan Heaps, research assistant, Woodrow Wilson School. The funding of this project came partly from a Ford Foundation Grant to the Woodrow Wilson School.

Information not otherwise credited in the text or referenced below is from the author's interviews and correspondence.

1. H. D. Laswell, Politics: Who Gets What, When, How, (McGraw Hill, New York, 1971).
2. N. Caplan and S. D. Nelson, "On Being Useful: The Nature and Consequences of Psychological Research on Social Problems," American Psychologist 28, 199-211 (1973).
3. I. Mitroff and R. O. Mason, "A Logic for Strategic Problem Solving: A Program of Research on Policy and Planning," Administrative Science Quarterly (forthcoming).
4. I. Mitroff and R. H. Kilman, Methodological Approaches to Social Sciences (Jossey-Bass, San Francisco, 1978), pp. 85-89.
5. At the July 12, 1977 Senate hearings, Mr. Ernst T. Krebs, Jr. specifically said that Laetrile is "Laevo-Mandelo-nitrile-beta-diglucoside."
6. FDA Consumer Memo, DHEW Publication No. (FDA)75-3007, n.d.
7. The 1962 amendments to the Food, Drug, and Cosmetic Act require that drugs introduced into interstate commerce be both safe and efficacious. To comply with this legislative requirement, the U.S. Food and Drug Administration (FDA) requires that all new drugs marketed after October 9, 1962, have an approved New Drug Application (NDA). In order to make application, pre-clinical testing of drugs prior to marketing is achieved through the sponsor submitting to FDA a notice of Claimed Investigational Exemption for a New Drug (IND). The IND consists of several phases following initial testing of animals.

Once studies conducted under the IND produce evidence
that the drug is safe and effective, the sponsor may submit an NDA. After an NDA is found to contain evidence
showing safety and effectiveness for a specific use, FDA
will approve it.

8.   U.S. Food and Drug Administration, Telegrams, In-House
     Memos, Testimony before State Legislatures (1976-79).

9.   R. F. Rich, Interviews with FDA Officials, State Offici-
     als, Proponents and Opponents of Laetrile (1978-79).

10. G. E. Markle, J. C. Petersen, and M. O. Wagenfeld, "Notes
     from the Cancer Underground: Participation in the Laet-
     rile Movement," Social Science and Medicine 12, 31-37.

11. R. Bradford, Statement to the U.S. Subcommittee on Health
     and Scientific Research (12 July 1977).

12. C. Friedrich, "Public Policy and the Nature of Adminis-
     trative Responsibility," pp. 414-425 in A. Altschuler
     (ed.), The Politics of Federal Bureaucracy, (Dodd, Mead
     and Co., New York, 1975).

13. H. Finer, "Administrative Responsibility in Democratic
     Government," pp. 425-432 in A. Altschuler (ed.), The
     Politics of Federal Bureaucracy (Dodd, Mead and Co.,
     New York, 1975).

5. The Laetrile Phenomenon: Legal Perspective

Conflicts in the legal philosophy of individual health care choices and the role of federal paternalism have emerged often in the courts. The tugging and pulling at the warp and woof of the legal system exerted by the Laetrile phenomenon's entry into the individual/federal rights thicket is nothing new in the health/cancer arena. The difference in the Laetrile proponents' successes appears to lie not with a real difference in issues but more with the learning process of the advocates and their ability to amass a verbal, supportive constituency. Theirs is a more sophisticated use of the judicial and legislative systems than their predecessors. Further, the appeal of their product -- Laetrile -- is not merely confined to the treatment of cancer. Rather, Laetrile is depicted not only as a drug but as a vitamin or food additive(1).

In this paper five topics are considered: federal drug regulation, informed consent, the right of privacy, physicians' rights and legal implications for cancer patients.

The underlying issue in the Laetrile case is the role of the federal government. The issue is, what kind of government do Americans want: a government that has responsibilities for protecting the consumers from vendors with worthless goods and services, a government that permits the strong to take advantage of the weak, a government that protects the consumer, or a government that sets standards and requires that all live up to those standards? To date, the majority speaking through the Congressional representatives has sought a government that protects the consumer and requires that vendors establish the value of their goods and follow an orderly process in distribution and selling. This process is reflected in the federal statutes regulating drugs. These statutes state that the caveat emptor doctrine is not applicable to the frightening and complex armament of

drugs for life-threatening illnesses. Viewed in this light,
federal drug legislation is merely part of a continuing consumer movement.

The emotional, scientific, legal and philosophic issues
related to Laetrile and cancer are tellingly stated by
Senator Edward Kennedy in his introductory remarks to the
Laetrile Hearings of 1977 (1, p. 1):

> The role of the Food and Drug Administration...
> is to guarantee that the available drug therapies
> are the best and most effective that science can
> devise. Their role is to protect both the patient
> and his family from remedies that are neither safe
> nor effective. The elimination of useless treat-
> ments is a valid Federal role. It is a humanatar-
> ian role. It reduces the burden on cancer patients
> and their families and allows them to exercise
> their freedom of choice on the basis of informed
> judgments among viable alternatives.

The Federal government, through the federal drug laws,
has made it clear that the manufacturers of all drugs must
prove their products safe and effective before they can be
offered to the consuming public. This congressional mandate,
which sets the first line of defense against ineffective
remedies, cannot be fulfilled on a discriminatory basis
where some remedies are banned as ineffective and others,
which have failed to meet identical scientific standards of
efficacy but have a dedicated pressure group behind them,
are allowed to be marketed. It is questionable whether the
congressional mandate can be a viable protection if partial
exemptions related to one class of consumer, the terminal
patient, are made. Discriminatory enforcement raises questions of the most serious kind relating to equal protection
of the laws, and exposes the entire regulatory apparatus to
ethical and legal assault.

There is no waffling in the intent of the federal drug
laws and regulations. They are to protect consumers, particularly those with life-threatening diseases who are prey
to fraudulent treatments. It is also clear from the judicial comment on the Act and its implementing regulations that
the tightening of regulations relating to drug safety and
efficacy paralleled the complexity of modern medicine and
medical practices (2). Federal drug regulation standards
require general recognition of safety and efficacy by experts in the treatment and research of the particular disease or condition studied and recognizes the hierarchy of
specialization which is a fact of scientific life. The

standards do not equate a general license to practice medicine with expertise in cancer research. The standards perceive that physician and consumer choices arise after the first cut is made -- after safety and efficacy of a product are reasonably established through expert recognition.

Is this congressional directive unwarranted paternalism? This is a political question. From the legal perspective, the Supreme Court, final judicial arbiter of our rights, has not so held.

Federal Drug Regulation

The Regulatory Plan

The Food, Drug, and Cosmetic Act (Act) (3), in conjunction with regulations promulgated by the Food and Drug Administration (FDA) pursuant to its statutory obligation to administer the Act, constitutes a comprehensive body of law governing the marketing of drugs for human or animal use intended to assure that drugs marketed in this country are both safe and effective. The FDA maintains that Laetrile is subject to the Act, while the Laetrile proponents have argued that Laetrile is not a drug, or that even if it is a drug, it is exempt.

Laetrile proponents have filed applications with the FDA. The John Beard Memorial Foundation filed a new drug application on October 3, 1962. However this application failed to provide data sufficient to demonstrate either the safety or efficacy of Laetrile and was declared incomplete by the FDA on February 25, 1963 (4). There is no indication that the John Beard Memorial Foundation came forth at that time with supplemental data adequate to cure the deficiencies in its application.

Again, in 1970 another attempt was made to obtain FDA sanction for the sale of Laetrile. This application was made by the McNaughton Foundation and sought an Investigational New Drug Exemption (IND) pursuant to Section 505(i) of the Act. The purpose of an IND is to allow a drug that has demonstrated its safety and efficacy in pre-clinical tests, for example, animal tests, to proceed to "investigational" testing on human subjects.

The FDA initially awarded the IND (No. 6734), but shortly thereafter, in the course of a routine review of the IND application, found serious problems with the applicant's clinical data. The FDA immediately requested that the applicant respond to two questions on manufacturing controls,

seven questions on pre-clinical tests and four medical
questions on data mentioned in the application but not
submitted. When the missing data were not provided by
McNaughton within the usual ten-day period allowed by the
FDA for the elimination of deficiencies, the IND was termin-
ated. It was not until some four months later that the
McNaughton Foundation responded to the FDA data request.

The FDA's action in terminating the Laetrile IND generated some Congressional interest. In response to this
interest, the FDA appointed a special committee of non-
government experts to review the entire Laetrile data file.
The committee found that independent laboratory assays provided no in vitro or in vivo evidence in animal models to
warrant trial of the substance in humans and thereby affirmed
the propriety of the FDA's action.

Critics of the FDA's Laetrile decision, specifically
Dean Burk, who at that time was on the National Cancer
Institute staff, and Andrew L. McNaughton, who was a party
to the application, had the opportunity to participate in
the committee's assessment. Rather than attempt to remedy
the deficiencies in the application pointed out by the special
committee, the Laetrile proponents never perfected their applications.

Two "grandfather" provisions are applicable to the Food,
Drug and Cosmetic Act and affect the need for a drug, which
otherwise is a "new drug," to comply with the pre-marketing
requirements of Section 505. The first of these grandfather
provisions is set forth in Section 201(p) itself and provides that notwithstanding the lack of general recognition
of safety and effectiveness, a drug shall not be declared
to be a "new drug"

> if at any time prior to the enactment of this
> chapter (June 25, 1938) it was subject to the
> Food and Drug Act of June 30, 1906, as amended,
> and if at such time its labeling contained in
> the same representations concerning the con-
> ditions of its use... (5).

The second grandfather exemption consists of the tran-
sitional provisions enacted as part of the 1962 amendments
of the Act, which states:

> In the case of any drug which, on the day
> immediately preceding the enactment date
> (October 10, 1962), (A) was commercially used
> or sold in the United States, (B) was not a

new drug as defined by Section 201(p) of the
basic Act as then in force and (C) was not
covered by an effective application under
Section 505 of the Act, the amendments of
Section 201(p) made by this Act shall not
apply to such drug when intended solely for
use under conditions prescribed, recommended
or suggested in labeling with respect to such
drug on that day (6).

The effect of the two grandfather clauses is to eliminate the requirement of obtaining an NDA for any drug subject
to the 1906 Act marketed in the United States from June 30,
1906, to June 25, 1938, or for any drug commercially used or
sold in the United States which in 1962 had attained general
recognition among qualified experts as safe for its intended
purpose, as the term "safe" was then properly interpreted
which for those with life-threatening illnesses included
efficacy (7, 26).

The elements required for general recognition of safety
are correctly stated by Commissioner Kennedy in the Laetrile
Rulemaking decision (8):

...for a drug to be generally recognized as safe it
must have accumulated at least the amount of evidence
of safety that would be required for the approval of
a new drug application and that evidence must be
generally available to the community of experts
through publication in the scientific literature.
In order for a new drug application for a drug to
be approved, there must exist as to that drug "adequate tests by all methods reasonably applicable"
that show the drug's safety.

Whether or not a drug is exempted from the pre-marketing
requirements of Section 505 by virtue of either of the above
grandfather clauses is to be determined initially by the FDA
(9). Additionally, it is incumbent upon the party seeking to
grandfather a drug to establish that the drug is in fact entitled to such status (10). The arguments presented to the
Rutherford court by the plaintiff cancer patient class is
that Laetrile falls within these grandfather exemptions (11).

Briefly stated, entitlement to the grandfather exemption
of the 1962 amendment, i.e., Section 197(c) (4) of the Food
and Drug Act, (6) which is the one found applicable by the
district court in Rutherford is limited to drugs which:
(1) feature today the identical chemical composition,
recommended dosages, and claims made in labeling as existed

on October 9, 1962, and; (2) were used or sold commercially in the United States on October 9, 1962, and; (3) were generally recognized by the experts as safe; and (4) were not covered by an effective new drug application (12).

Laetrile and Federal Enforcement Actions

In 1960 the FDA began the first in a continuing series of enforcement actions with the seizure of Laetrile in Dallas. These actions have generally been decided promptly in favor of the FDA based on the finding that Laetrile is not generally recognized as safe and effective and has not been approved for marketing (13). Recent enforcement actions have also included the seizure of interstate shipments of apricot kernels destined for use in the manufacture of Laetrile (14).

As in many studies, it is the exceptional case which provides the best medium for analysis. In the Laetrile controversy that exception is Rutherford v. United States (15). Rutherford was instituted by cancer patients in the United States District Court for the Western District of Oklahoma on March 12, 1975 (16). The suit sought to prevent the government from interfering with the sale and distribution of Laetrile by obtaining a decree which would preclude the government from conducting seizure, injunctive or criminal actions against Laetrile and its proponents. The district court entered an order which permitted Mr. Rutherford to obtain a limited quantity of Laetrile. The government sought review of this order before the United States Court of Appeals for the Tenth Circuit in Denver. The Tenth Circuit directed that the case be remanded to the FDA for the development of an administrative record on whether Laetrile is a "new drug," and if so, whether it is exempt from the pre-marketing approval requirements of the Act (18).

In rendering this opinion, the Tenth Circuit made two significant findings -- one in accord and one not in accord with the Act.

Before determining whether Laetrile was a "new drug" it was necessary for the Appeals Court to decide whether it was a drug under the Act. The Laetrile proponents had argued that Laetrile was a Vitamin, a dietary supplement, or a naturally occurring food, but that it was not a drug. The court found, however, that Laetrile was "unquestionably" intended as a treatment for cancer, and that even if it is a food, it is also a drug subject to the Act because it is intended for use in the cure, mitigation, treatment, or prevention of cancer (15, p. 11, n. 2). This decision was

in accord with both the legislative history of the Act and
a well-established body of case law indicating that it is
the intended use of a substance which determines whether a
product is considered a food, a drug, or both under the
regulatory plan (17).

The holding not in accord with the Act deals with standards and burden of proof. The court of appeals and the
district court below, from the outset, have eschewed the
statutory standard and have created a hybrid standard which
literally requires the FDA to initiate an administrative
proceeding on drug status and bear the burden of proof in
that proceeding at anytime the FDA has stated that a product
is a "new drug" but doesn't have an administrative record,
opinion or application to point to in substantiation of its
statement:

> We are unable, however, to see how the FDA
> can escape the obligation of producing an admin-
> istrative record to support its determination of
> the first and more fundamental issue that Laetrile
> is a new drug, for it is not a new drug merely
> because they say it is ... To support its deter-
> mination the FDA in the case at bar would have to
> present substantial evidence to support the propo-
> sition that Laetrile is not generally recognized
> among qualified experts as "safe and effective,"
> and that Laetrile is not grandfathered by either
> of the exemptions discussed above (18).

The FDA is not required by any provision in the federal
drug laws or any principle of administrative law to initiate
a rulemaking proceeding to determine the "new drug" or
"grandfather" status of a product before the agency can
declare that product to be a "new drug." Further, Judge
Kiley, in Tutoki v. Celebrezze (19), denying declaratory
relief against the FDA to cancer patients seeking Krebiozen
for failure to exhaust their administrative remedies express-
ly found that the statute did not preclude cancer patients
from sponsoring an NDA for Krebiozen. Finally, Judge
Hastings speaking for a unanimous court in Rutherford v.
American Medical Association et al. (20), as one basis for
his decision denying an injunction against the FDA requiring
it to cease interfering with patient/physician procurement
of Krebiozen, held that the Krebiozen proponents had not
shown that they had made a good faith attempt to comply with
the procedures established by Congress for the introduction
of new drugs.

Thus in a number of cases parallel to Rutherford, courts

have held that they would permit no dilution of the standards
and procedures for determination of the status of a drug if
the proponent position was shifted from manufacturer/
developer to patient. Deviation from the prescribed statutory standard of proof is also inconsistent with the positions of the parties in Rutherford. The "evidence" which
the FDA is supposed to provide lies within in the control of
those physicians and manufacturers who are said to be using
and making Laetrile. This process can "require" the production of evidence.

The administrative proceedings required by Judge Bohanon
produced over 400 written submissions, comprising some 5,500
pages of material, and included two days of public hearings.
The submissions represented a broad spectrum of views from
cancer patients, consumers, experts in drug testing and
cancer therapy, physicians, state governments, universities,
hospitals, and organizations such as the American Cancer
Society and the Committee for Freedom of Choice in Cancer
Therapy. It is upon this body of information that the Commissioner of the Food and Drug Administration based his
decision. The Commissioner found that Laetrile did not
qualify for exemption under either of the grandfather
clauses. He concluded that Laetrile was not exempt from
the safety and effectiveness requirements under the 1938
grandfather clause because there was "no proof submitted to
show that what was termed 'Laetrile' or 'amygdalin' as used
before 1938 was the same drug which is now being marketed
..." and that there is no "indication whatever that the
labeling ... before 1938 contained representations concerning conditions of use which are identical to the representations associated with the presently marketed drug" (8, p.
39788).

Laetrile did not qualify for exemption under the 1962
grandfather because, first, the composition of the drug
presently referred to as Laetrile was not shown to be the
same as the drug used during the grandfather period. Second,
Laetrile was not commercially used or sold in the United
States on the grandfather date. This conclusion is supported
by the new drug application filed by proponents of Laetrile
on October 3, 1962. The drug had previously been shipped
for investigational and not commercial purposes, as Dr.
Krebs, Sr. indicated, and a June 1962 court order, entered
following the conviction of Mr. Krebs, Jr., for violating the
new drug provisions of the Act, substantiates this. The new
drug application itself indicates that the drug was not
commercially available for use (8, p. 39779).

The third basis for denying the 1962 grandfather exemp-

tion was the lack of information concerning the labeled conditions of use on the grandfather date. No labeling was
described or submitted for a product in use on the grandfather date, and labeling proposed for use and in use before
and after the grandfather date were not similar. Finally,
the Commissioner found that on the grandfather date, experts
did not recognize Laetrile as safe for use under any conditions since they were largely unfamiliar with the drug,
lacked information as to its composition and labeled conditions of use, and, in the absence of any published literature
reporting results of tests which showed the drug to be safe
or effective, had no basis in scientific data upon which to
recognize the drug as safe (8, p. 39792-5).

The district court then reviewed the Commissioner's
decision. In reviewing administrative decisions the court's
duty is only to decide whether the agency has acted arbitrar-
ily, or in abuse of its discretion. The district court characterized the administrative record as revealing "a substantial and well-developed controversy among medical professionals and other scientists as to the efficacy of Laetrile," and
accepted the Commissioner's conclusion that Laetrile is not
generally recognized as safe and effective. Similarly, the
court sustained the Commissioner's denial of an exemption
for Laetrile based on the 1938 grandfather clause (21).

The district court concluded, however, that Laetrile
was exempt under the 1962 grandfather clause. In reaching
this conclusion the district court rejected each of the
Commissioner's factual findings. The district court found
that Laetrile is identical to amygdalin and has had a con-
tinuous identical composition, that the availability of
amygdalin from chemical supply houses establishes the commercial availability of Laetrile as a pharmaceutical product,
that the labeling for Laetrile was established by a new drug
application filed in October 1962 and that Laetrile was
generally recognized as safe prior to the grandfather date.

In reaching its decision the district court virtually
ignored the evidence relied upon by the Commissioner to
support his findings and simply cited other evidence. Such
a re-weighing of evidence was improper. The district court
also held that by denying the right to use a nontoxic substance in connection with one's own personal health-care,
FDA has offended the constitutional right to privacy (15).

The decision of the district court was reviewed by the
United States Court of Appeals of the Tenth Circuit. Rather
surprisingly, the court of appeals did not explicitly
address the statutory or constitutional issues on which the

district court decided the case. Rather, in a short opinion
unsupported by citation of authority or the record, the
court of appeals held that the "safety" and "effectiveness"
requirements of the Act have no application to terminally
ill cancer patients who desire to take Laetrile intravenously. The FDA, in the court's opinion, had not advanced a
standard against which to measure the safety and effectiveness of Laetrile as applied to such plaintiffs (22).

The court emphasized that its opinion is strictly
limited to terminally ill cancer patients and the intravenous use of Laetrile. A certificate by a licensed medical
practitioner that a particular person is terminally ill with
cancer was considered sufficient although "terminal" was
left undefined. The court did not mention the use of
Laetrile in tablet form or explain why it restricted usage to
intravenous administration. The FDA was left to "promulgate
regulations within the above limitations as if the drug was
found by the Commission (sic) to be 'safe' and 'effective'
for the limited group of persons here considered" (22, p. 6).
Rutherford's later request to allow the oral use of Laetrile
was denied by the court without comment (23).

The decision of the court of appeals broke new ground
when it flatly declared that the safety and efficacy provisions of the Act were inapplicable to Laetrile administered
intravenously by a physician to terminally ill cancer
patients. There is no basis in the language of the statute
or the legislative history which supports an exception for
terminally ill cancer patients. The essential purpose of
the Act is to ensure that all available drugs are both safe
and effective for their intended uses (26).

While the court of appeals held the statutory criteria
of safety and efficacy inapplicable, it employed two separate safety criteria and misconstrued the meaning of efficacy
in formulating its opinion. First, it required that the
drug be administered by a physician; that is a criteria of
safety embodied in the Act (24). Second, the court of
appeals limited its holding to intravenous administration;
it did not deem orally administered Laetrile to be within
the exception it created. This distinction is unexplained.
While neither oral or intravenous administration have been
systematically studied, the court recognized by implication
that oral administration may result in cyanide poisoning.
The effects of intravenous administration are more uncertain.

The holding of the Court of Appeals that "effective"
has no meaning if the person by all prevailing standards is
going to die of cancer regardless of what may be done is too

narrow in terms of the class it addresses -- the terminally
ill. Where a cure may not be possible, other relief for the
terminally ill may be, for example, pain control, appetite
stimulation, odor reduction, tranquilization. Under the
circumstances, where the current thrust of the Laetrile proponents seems to be that it will dramatically relieve pain,
improve appetite, promote weight gain, reduce the odor associated with cancer, improve the cancer patient's general
sense of well-being, control or prevent cancer, it would seem
logical that the terminally ill are entitled to the assurance
that the products they seek to use are effective when measured against the claims of sponsor.

Furthermore, the court of appeals assumes that an objective standard is available or can be formulated and
applied to determine who is "terminally ill." This assumption is in conflict with the findings made by the Commissioner in the Laetrile decision. The thrust of those findings
is that cancer is a disease that affects individual patients
and that physicians dealing with these patients on an individual basis find it difficult to distinguish the in-fact
terminal from non-terminal cancer patients with any accuracy.
The practical and ethical problems of carving out an exception for the terminally ill from the Act was pointedly
addressed by Dr. Samuel Klagsbrun:

> Use of the term "terminally ill" is inappro-
> priate when dealing with an individual cancer
> patient. Although specific forms of cancer may
> have a statistically expectable mortality rate,
> that rate is meaningless when applied to an
> individual patient. Oncologists are all familiar
> with experiences where severe cancers, which were
> statistically considered to be hopeless, have, in
> some small percentages of cases, undergone a sudden
> remission. It would be tragic to condemn any indi-
> vidual cancer patient to death because, as a
> statistical matter, that patient's particular form
> of cancer may not be curable.

> A decision to allow patients who are diagnosed
> as having a cancer which, as a statistical matter is
> expected to lead to their death, would move all such
> patients away from orthodox therapy and condemn even
> the individual patient whose cancer may unexpectedly
> move into remission to Laetrile, a worthless and in-
> effective drug. In addition, such a decision would
> thereafter remove the patients from the possibility
> of receiving continuing chemotherapy or radiation
> therapy which could enhance the effects of any

remission. Most physicians have undergone the
experience of predicting the moment of death
and have been unexpectedly and repeatedly
proven wrong to a considerable degree. The
prolongation of life, therefore, becomes a
goal, not simply for the sake of prolongation,
but also to render patients available to either
a recent advance in chemotherapy or simply to
enhance the quality of the time left available
to the patients (25).

The government asked the Supreme Court to review the
decision in the Rutherford case. Review was granted on
January 22, 1979. The issues which were presented for review and briefed to the Court are the application of the
federal drug laws to the terminal and also the alternative
grounds for decision presented in the district court
opinion -- the grandfather exemption and the right of privacy.

On June 18, 1979 the Supreme Court issued its decision
on Laetrile (26). The Court did not address the constitutional and grandfather clause issues. It confined its
opinion to the terminal exception created by the Tenth
Circuit. The bottom line of the Supreme Court's decision
is that the rationale for the 10th Circuit's opinion is
unsupportable, that there is nothing in the congressional
history or administrative interpretation of the federal
drug laws that supports an exemption for the terminally ill.
Further, as the Court explains at length, the inclusion of
the terminal within the coverage of the Act, is reasonably
related to the Act's purposes as the Court perceives them.
The Court thus reversed the 10th Circuit and remanded the
case for further proceedings consistent with its opinion.
These further proceedings mean that the 10th Circuit should
now look at the grounds for decision articulated by the
district court (grandfather clause/constitution) which it
did not deal with in its opinion and issue an opinion dealing with the bases upon which the district court reached
its decision.

The key points of the Court's decision are:

The federal drug laws make no express exemption for
drugs used by the terminally ill.

    (1) No implicit exemption is necessary to attain
         congressional objectives (26, p. 7):
         (a) Legislative history indicates that Congress
            was concerned with the protection of those

with fatal illnesses (<u>26</u>, pp. 7-8).

(b) The administrative authority implementing
the federal drug laws (FDA) in its application and interpretation of the Act has
not made an exemption for drugs used for
the terminal or those with life-threatening
illness.

(c) Congress was aware of the FDA's interpretation of the Act and approved of it (1962
Amendments & Reports).

(d) The history of purportedly simple and painless cancer cures suggests why Congress
could "reasonably have determined to
protect the terminally ill, no less than
other patients, from the vast range of
self-styled panaceas that inventive minds
can devise" (<u>26</u>, p. 13).

(2) <u>An implicit exemption is not necessary to avert</u>
<u>an unreasonable reading of the terms "safe" and</u>
<u>"effective."</u>

<u>Congress could reasonably have intended to shield</u>
<u>terminal patients from ineffectual or unsafe drugs</u> (<u>26</u>,
p. 10).

(a) Effectiveness does not necessarily mean
capacity to cure, it also extends to a
sponsor's claims of prolonged life, improved physical condition or reduced pain.

(b) Safety does have meaning for the terminal.
A drug is unsafe for the terminal, as for
anyone else, if its potential for inflict-
ing death or physical injury is not offset
by the possibility of therapeutic benefit.
The 10th Circuit implicitly acknowledged
safety as a factor by restricting Laetrile
to IV use.

(c) Safety/efficacy have a special meaning in
the context of incurable illness: "if an
individual suffering from a potentially
fatal disease rejects conventional therapy
in favor of a drug with no demonstrable
curative properties, the consequences can
be irreversible" (<u>26</u>, p. 11). This
special meaning is supported by FDA administrative interpretation and by expert
testimony in the record.

(d) Experimental drugs are available for the
terminal for whom conventional treatment
is unavailing through special FDA procedures.

The Supreme Court's decision removes only part of the cloud in federal regulation of interstate Laetrile posed by the Rutherford decision. Since the legal access to Laetrile by cancer patients lies through the affidavit process in the Rutherford court and that access could be sustained by a finding that there is a constitutional right to use Laetrile or that it is grandfathered, the full reach of federal authority will remain unclear until the 10th Circuit's opinion on remand and possible further action by the Supreme Court. However, language in the Supreme Court's opinion on the federal interest in regulation of drugs for those with life threatening illness signals that the Court would not look favorably on a constitutional right of privacy as applied to ineffective drugs. Further, the confused history of the formula, recommended use and administration of Laetrile prior to 1962 set forth in the Commissioners' decision and briefed to the Supreme Court (27) in Rutherford likewise signals that this rationale for Laetrile access will not stand close judicial scrutiny.

Interplay of Federal and State Statutes

State statutes legitimating the marketing of Laetrile have had little actual effect due to the lack of raw materials, such as apricot kernels in the state. Interstate shipment of apricot kernels or other raw materials intended for use in manufacture of Laetrile is prohibited by the federal Act for it reaches interstate shipment of the major components or active ingredients of a drug. Similarly, a drug manufactured and distributed solely within one state is still subject to the federal Act as its main component was shipped in interstate commerce. The state statutes that have approved Laetrile do constitute an important statement of either pro-Laetrile or anti-government sentiment.

Although the issue has not been litigated, the validity of state regulation in the face of federal prohibition may be questioned. Under the supremacy clause of the federal constitution where "Congress has taken the particular subject matter in hand," the states are precluded from regulating that same "subject matter" (28). Where preemption occurs, all state regulation is invalid.

In the context of the Laetrile controversy, it can be argued that the federal Act, which requires safety and effectiveness, by its very nature demands national uniformity of a virtually absolute character. A federal Act which regulates drugs in all states except those which prefer otherwise may be deemed incompatible with the notion of pro-

viding effective protection against unsafe and ineffective
drugs. The legislative history of the federal Act also indicates a Congressional intent that the Act establish uniform
drug standards (29). The question then becomes whether the
state statutes exempting Laetrile do so in a manner violative
of the federal requirements of uniformity. Under the circumstances it is not unreasonable to contend that it does although the answer is not clear. Finally, a number of the
Laetrile statutes specifically provide that the state board
of health or pharmacy may set standards to assure that the
substance is not adulterated, misbranded or otherwise contaminated (30). If these provisions are not being enforced,
enforcement could be mandated through administrative action.

What of those states that do not specifically provide
for adulteration/misbranding control? Are the guidelines or
the state drug laws requiring procedures to assure that
drugs sold within the state are neither adulterated nor misbranded automatically written into the Laetrile statutes?
This question can only be answered by direct inquiry to the
various Attorneys General. If the answer is negative, there
is a serious question of danger to the public health. This
danger may support a federal pre-emption argument.

The Informed Consent and Physician Liability Issues

The right to bodily control has its expression in the
doctrine of informed consent which is a key element in the
federal district court cases which have permitted Laetrile
treatment to cancer patients and also in a number of statutes
legalizing Laetrile.

By way of illustration, a Rutherford informed consent
form requires a physician's declaration that the patient is
terminally ill; 1. that there is histologic evidence of a
rapidly progressive malignancy in the patient possessive of
a high and predictable mortality rate; and 2. either (a) that
further orthodox treatment would not reasonably be expected
to benefit the patient; or (b) that Laetrile will be administered only in conjunction with established and recognized
forms of cancer treatment; or (c) that the patient has made
a knowing and intelligent election to take Laetrile after
being fully apprised of the full range of recognized treatments available and of the fact that Laetrile is considered
by most cancer experts to be of no value in combatting the
disease. In comparison, the Indiana statute legalizing
Laetrile contains a consent form which requires a physician's
explanation to patient that the manufacture and distribution
of Laetrile is banned by FDA; that it is not a recommended

treatment and that there are alternative recognized treatments for that patient's cancer (31).

To assure the level of protection from liability provided by the federal informed consent procedure and required in the case law involving informed consent (32), it would appear that the physician confronted with a patient desiring treatment by Laetrile, should augment the sample statutory or court forms with the traditional elements of informed consent omitted from those forms. Without such protective augmentation, the subjective intent of the patient becomes material. In methods of treatment not yet accepted by the medical professional generally, where the contemplated therapeutic benefits are unknown or speculative, the facts as known or unknown to the attending physician are of material importance to the patient/subject's decision. Does the patient/subject perceive Laetrile as a cure, a pain reliever, a control for cancer, a preventative agent, an appetite stimulant, an aid to the removal of the odor of decaying tumor tissue, a mood elevator? Does the physician represent his utilization of the substance as meeting any of the above conditions?

The Laetrile informed consent issue presents problems not usually confronted in the jurisprudence of informed consent. It is a product which is generally considered by experts in the field of cancer research and treatment as ineffective and unproven after over 20 years in the medical arena. This compares with chemotherapeutic agents which may be of medically recent origin, but which emanate from research centers with reputations which bear out a track record for effective treatment and for which informed consent for human experimentation procedures are a commonplace and crucial part of day-to-day practice.

If the consent procedure has included a clear statement of the elements of treatment and possible outcome, for example, palliate not cure, and the patient consents because he believes the substance will cure, the physician is not responsible if the patient's expectations are not fulfilled. However, what if both the physician and the patient are believers in Laetrile. What if the physician takes the position that the informed consent requirement imposed by the state legislature is merely a nuisance restriction and is meaningless? The physician informs the patient as stated on the sample forms of the non-therapeutic expectations attributable to Laetrile by the general expert medical community but by his own attitudes and remarks reinforces the patient's belief in the cure, prevention or control of the disease by Laetrile. What then?

If the physician-patient contract contains a promise of cure, is the informed consent form which represents that the cure is not a reasonably anticipated benefit of the treatment a nullity? Is the physician then liable for breach of a contract for cure (33)? Further, is a physician who either intentionally or negligently misrepresents the nature or results of treatment he has rendered liable for fraud? There is authority that answers this question in the affirmative (34).

Indeed, can any consent system that operates on the principle that the drug is ineffective have legitimacy when the only reason the placebo effect of a drug works is because the recipient believes the drug to be effective? Placebo effect is described by Dan Martin, M.D. in the Laetrile Rulemaking proceeding as "a form of self-hypnosis based on the power of positive thinking." The underlying assumption by the district court and the court of appeals that the substance is ineffective but it does not matter if the patients know that and still want it, is false. The patients would not be seeking the drug if they did not believe it effective.

Finally, what type of recovery will be available to patients, or protection available to physicians if the patterns followed in Nevada and Oklahoma become the rule? In Oklahoma, the law requires patients to agree to waive malpractice suits if Laetrile is prescribed at their request. Nevada Medical Liability Insurance Association which writes 60% of state malpractice suits won't extend malpractice coverage to Laetrile suits. Further, with regard to physician liability, most of the statutes passed by the states that deal with "Laetrile/amygdalin" do not (35) legalize its sale or distribution (36). Most statutes merely affect a physician's use of Laetrile in two very limited ways: (a) prohibiting hospital and health facilities from interfering in the doctor/patient relationship by restricting or forbidding the use of the substance when prescribed or administered by a physician and requested by a patient and (b) prohibiting disciplinary action against a physician who prescribes or administers the substance upon patient request.

Some of these statutes have a criterion which provides a way of effectively nullifying the state statute without further legislative action. I refer to provisions for a hearing by a state medical board to determine if the substance is harmful (37). Once found "harmful," the physician would no longer be covered by the umbrella protection from hospital or health facility interference with his administration of Laetrile or from disciplinary action (30).

According to the Alaska Attorney General, statutes which merely preclude hospital interference or physician discipline may fairly be interpreted as not removing physicians from liability under the states pure drug laws. Under his interpretation, state drug laws which prohibit sale, delivery or "give away" of drugs that are not found safe or effective would still apply to the physician. Thus, in its most liberal interpretation, a physician merely prescribing Laetrile or administering the Laetrile delivered to him by the patient may not be subject to state drug law strictures, but the physician who sells or gives away Laetrile would be (**30**).

The Right of Privacy

Warner V. Slack, writing in "Points of View" (**38**) places the physician/patient decision-making issue in perspective helpful to exploration of why the right of privacy concept has emerged as central to the legal aspects of the Laetrile phenomenon. Dr. Slack observes that:

> For centuries, the medical profession has perpetrated paternalism as an essential component of medical care and thereby deprived patients of the self-esteem that comes from self-reliance. "I believe that the loss of decision-making is probably the heaviest blow of all to most patients' morale," wrote J.L.W. Price after a stay in the hospital. It seems to be that patients will be more likely to adhere to treatment regimens when they can make their own decisions and that, given the opportunity, more and more patients will elect to do so.

These perceptions seem to track the psychology of the Laetrile phenomenon. They relate to a concept which touches a strong cord both in the American way of life and in American jurisprudence and encompass the historical concept of control over one's person and destiny: "Outside areas of plainly harmful conduct, every American is left to shape his own life as he thinks best, do what he pleases, go where he pleases" (**39**). This quotation from a Justice Douglas' Supreme Court concurring opinion is relied upon by United States District Court Judge Luther Bohanon in his opinion in Rutherford v. United States, to support the right of actual or supposed cancer patients to procure and utilize Laetrile. The keystones of the Judge Bohanon decision are dealt with in detail in the following sections; in brief, they are:

1) Freedom to care for one's health and person comes within the purview of the right of privacy guaranteed by the Constitution.

2) Implicit in the right of privacy is the right "to be let alone."

3) The right of privacy includes the privilege of an individual to plan his own affairs, for "outside areas of plainly harmful conduct, every American is left to shape his own life as he thinks best, to do what he pleases, go where he pleases."

4) A patient has the right to refuse cancer treatment altogether, therefore, he has a further right, should he decide to forego conventional treatment, to enlist such non-toxic treatment, however unconventional, as he finds to be of comfort--particularly where recommended by his physician.

These concepts are also expressed in the appeals court decision in the Privitera case (40) which involved the rights of physicians to assert a patient's right to privacy as a defense to statutory of medical board prohibitions against a physician administering a treatment not regarded as safe and effective by qualified experts: (1) every human being of adult years and sound mind has a right to determine what shall be done with his own body, (2) the right to control one's own body is not restricted to the wise; it includes the "foolish" refusal of medical treatment (41), (3) the right to choose what may be a suicidal medical course has been upheld (42), and (4) Roe dealt specifically with the right to determine one's own medical treatment. Another element of the right of privacy arguments focused on in Privitera is informed consent: "Where informed consent is adequately insured, there is no justification for infringing upon the patient's right to privacy in selecting and con-senting to the treatment" (43).

In holding that a right of privacy related to health care does exist and is applicable to the drug Laetrile, Judge Bohanon in Rutherford cites Justice Douglas' concurring opinion in the Roe and Doe cases (39). Justice Douglas con-tended that many rights not specifically enumerated in the Constitution come within the meaning of the term liberty as used in the Fourteenth Amendment. After listing (1) control over the development and expression of one's intellect, interests, tastes and personality and (2) the freedom of choice in the basic decisions of one's life respecting marriage, divorce, procreation, contraception and the educa-tion and upbringing of children, Justice Douglas notes (3) the freedom to care for one's health and person, freedom from bodily restraint or compulsion, freedom to walk, stroll,

or lope as coming, in his view, within the meaning of the
term, "liberty."

Judge Bohanon relied upon Justice Douglas' discussion
of his second group of freedoms (44), rather than in the
third group of freedoms which ostensibly deal with health.
After asserting that this third group of rights are fundamental and subject to regulation only upon a showing of
compelling state interest, Justice Douglas does not cite
cases to the effect that freedom to care for one's health as
opposed to freedom from bodily restraint or compulsion or
freedom to work, stroll or lope, are fundamental rights
subject to strict judicial scrutiny under the Constitution.
The discussion following this third group of rights concerns
freedom from bodily restraint, freedom of movement, and protection pursuant to the Fourth Amendment from governmental
intrusions. The concept of health care is not delineated or
defined. Furthermore, Justice Douglas was not joined by any
other Justice in his concurring opinion and the Court's later
characterization of these cases markedly differs from that
suggested by Justice Douglas.

The Supreme Court has specifically indicated that the
rational basis or reasonable means test should be applied
where the validity of legislation such as the new drug
safety and effectiveness standards established by the Act is
at issue. In Whalen v. Roe, the Court upheld a state statute requiring that identification of the prescribing physician and patient be prepared and filed with the state whenever a "Schedule II" drug (45) is prescribed. The court held
that the constitutional right of privacy did not attach to the
decision to use Schedule II drugs, even though the disclosure
requirements would [u]nquestionably ... lead some patients
to avoid or postpone needed medical attention" (46, p. 602).
The constitutionality of regulation was based on a rational
relationship test and not on the compelling state interest
standard. The Court also indicated that the state could prohibit entirely the use of a particular Schedule II drug
despite its medically recognized use. It would seem, therefore, that if a state may ban a drug which has a recognized
medical use, its authority to ban a drug such as Laetrile,
which has no recognized medical use, is beyond question.

The conclusion that the United States Supreme Court has
not recognized a right of privacy in the case of medical
treatment choices involving drugs was the keystone of the
California Supreme Court's decision which overturned the
state appeals court rationale opening the door to Laetrile
access (47). In that opinion the Supreme Court of California speaking through Judge Clark rejected the argument of

Dr. Privitera and his attorney that there is a fundamental right protected by the federal and California constitutions to obtain Laetrile. The court held that since no fundamental right is involved, the appropriate standard of review is the rationale basis test, that is, is there a reasonable relationship of the regulation to legitimate state interests in health and safety of its citizens rather than the compelling state interest test.

The history of cancer therapy in this country illustrates the justification for Government concern that, absent pre-marketing clearance, useless drugs will flourish. As the Commission found in the Laetrile Decision, there has been a long and sorry history of cancer quackery, during which "literally thousands of supposed remedies for cancer" have been promoted (8, pp. 39795-97). As the Commissioner found in the Laetrile Decision, promoters of worthless cancer remedies are often particularly successful because of the fear engendered by the disease, and the modest hope offered by legitimate remedies. The cancer patient wants to believe that there is a painless, effective remedy. The "placebo" effect of Laetrile, if any, is achieved only because the cancer victim is successfully deceived into believing that the drug will be effective.

The district court in Rutherford suggests that the exemption of Laetrile from the Act "in no way portends the return of the traveling snake oil salesman ... FDA is fully empowered under other statutory provisions to combat false or fraudulent advertising of ineffectual or unproven drugs." However, the suggestion that the FDA will be able to adequately police the claims of drug promoters, absent a system of pre-marketing clearance, is wholly unrealistic and bereft of any supportive findings or analysis. The crisis this country faces in environmental and industrial pollutants is one example of what the absence of pre-marketing clearance can produce.

The Food and Drug Administration's authority to control misbranding applies only to false or misleading claims made in a drug's "labeling." "Labeling" refers to matter which accompanies the drugs. FDA would be unable to control claims made for Laetrile, or other drugs, in books, pamphlets, and oral communications which do not "accompany" or which cannot otherwise be linked to the drug. Moreover, by forcing the FDA to prove that a drug is misbranded, the district court in Rutherford has reversed the burden of proof intended by Congress. As the House Committee noted, the FDA, with its limited resources, would be required to amass the scientific material necessary to prove that each fraudulent drug is

ineffective. Promoters of the drug would be able to market
it, and reap the profits, pending investigation and litaga-
tion. Congress' determination that fraudulent remedies can
only be effectively barred from the market by forcing the
manufacturer to assume the burden of proving effectiveness
is entirely reasonable.

In the case of cancer, a significant number of patients
can be cured, or permitted to live normal lives longer, by
legitimate therapy, especially if treatment is begun early.
The record in the Laetrile Decision proceeding before the
FDA indicates that the availability of Laetrile serves to
encourage delay in obtaining such legitimate therapy, or
avoidance of such therapy altogether. The Supreme Court in
its Rutherford opinion recognizes the danger an ineffective
drug poses to the patient with a life threatening illness:

> "But if an individual suffering from a
> potentially fatal disease rejects conven-
> tional therapy in favor of a drug with no
> demonstrable curative properties, the con-
> sequences can be irreversible" (48).

Moreover, even among patients who begin treatment with effective therapy, the readily acknowledged side effects and
hazards of that therapy may cause them to abandon such
methods at a time when their application might still be beneficial, and to turn instead to Laetrile, a "painless cure."
The drug's promoters actively encourage this process, playing
on the cancer victims' fears. Particularly in the case of
cancer which inspires fear in victims, the only means of
preventing patients from being drawn to the simple, fraudulent cures is to ban them from the market.

The Rutherford district court noted that most persons
taking Laetrile probably know that the government and most
experts consider it worthless. The court did not discuss,
however, the FDA Commissioner's findings that the psychological pressures and fears of cancer victims and their
families leave them in a position where emotion may overrule
intellect. The district court suggests no means by which
those who are psychologically incapable of making an objective decision about Laetrile, or any other remedy promoted
for a serious disease, may be distinguished from those who
are susceptible to being misled by alluring claims of a
quick and easy cure.

Physicians' Rights: The Privitera Case

Section 1707.1 of the California Health and Safety Code

requires the pre-marketing clearance of a drug used in connection with cancer -- to wit, a drug must be approved either
by the state board as safe and effective, or by the FDA pursuant to Section 505 of the Food, Drug and Cosmetic Act which
requires proof of safety and effectiveness. The state and
federal statutes contain nearly identical language requiring
"full reports of investigations which have been made to show
whether or not such drug is safe for use and whether such
drug is effective in use..."

The Privitera appeals court (49) found in general that
the purpose of the California statute which it stated as
frustrating cancer quacks and promoting early and effective
care of cancer is not served by prohibiting a licensed doctor
from giving an unapproved drug. With specific reference to
physicians' rights, the court agreed with the arguments of
Dr. Privitera who was convicted of a felony, conspiracy to
sell, prescribe an unapproved drug intended for the alleviation or cure of cancer -- that a patient's constitutionally
grounded right of privacy to use Laetrile therapy extends
to physicians willing to administer the drug and to suppliers
of that drug and further, that physicians possess an independent right to practice medicine generally and to prescribe
medicine and to use procedures without unreasonable government intervention.

The derivative right argument is completely addressed
by the Supreme Court in Whalen v. Roe (46, p. 604) "...the
doctor's claim is derivative from, and therefore no stronger
than, the patient's. Our rejection of their claim there
disposes of the doctor's as well." If there is a compelling
state interest in precluding the choice of treatments involving unsafe or ineffective drugs for cancer -- there is
then no right to choose in the patient and no derivative
right in the physician. Therein, contrasted against the
Supreme Court's holdings, lies one error of the Privitera
court.

The error was addressed and corrected by the highest
court of the state of California in an opinion issued on
March 15, 1979 (47). The principles underpinning that
court's refusal to recognize a patient's right of privacy
and a derivative physician right are as follows:

The United States Supreme Court has not recognized a
right of privacy in the case of medical treatment. The
court indicated that several Supreme Court cases present
lessons that are applicable to the California Supreme Court's
deliberation.

Roe v. Wade (39) upheld the regulation of abortion procedure locations and appropriate personnel by the state,
applying the rationale basis test. The specific application
of this case to the Supreme Court of California's delibera-
tions are stated as follows by Justice Clark: "A requirement
that a drug be certified effective for its intended use is a
reasonable means to 'insure maximum safety for the patient'."

The Supreme Court of California discussed the decision
of Planned Parenthood v. Danforth (50) and the assistance it
was to their decision as follows. The decision to be treated
(have an abortion) "may be within the constitutional zone of
privacy deserving the protection provided by the compelling
interest standard, the selection of a particular procedure is
a medical matter to which privacy status does not attach and
which may be regulated by the government, providing a rational
basis for such regulation exists."

Whalen v. Roe (46) dealt with controlled substances.
The Court characterized the importance of this case to its
decision as follows: "If the state has the power to ban a
drug with a recognized medical use because of its potential
for abuse, then - given a rationale basis for doing so - the
state clearly has the power to ban a drug not recognized as
effective for its intended use."

The Supreme Court of California found that the statute
satisfies the rational relationship test.

Judge Clark speaking for the Court found that California's legitimate state interest was set forth in Section 1700
of its state statute which expressed the state's concern with
the effective and early diagnosis, and treatment or the cure
of persons suffering from cancer.

In further support of the finding that the rationale
relationship test was fulfilled, the Court cited the Commissioner's rulemaking decision in the Laetrile proceeding, and
specifically the Commissioner's finding that Laetrile is not
generally recognized as a safe and effective cancer drug and
does not qualify for an exemption from the Food, Drug and
Cosmetic Act under the Grandfather clause.

The Supreme Court of California discussed and held inapplicable the exemption of the terminally ill from coverage
of the Federal Drug Laws as was done in the Rutherford
opinion.

The Supreme Court of California discussed the Ruther-

ford v. United States Court of Appeals decision which was
entered by the Tenth Circuit on July 10, 1978. The Court
held this decision inapplicable in the California forum because (1) there is "no indication in the record that the
defendant's (physician) sought to restrict their activities
to that class of patients." In addition, Judge Clark noted
that "Dr. Privitera sometimes took neither a medical history
from or personally examined the patients for whom he prescribed Laetrile. The lay defendants, of course, were not
qualified to diagnose cancer, much less to determine whether
a cancerous condition was 'terminal'." (2) the Commissioner's refusal to approve Laetrile for terminal patients in
the Laetrile rulemaking proceedings was reasonable and
supported by substantial evidence; and (3) the record in the
California proceeding does not inspire confidence that
Laetrile advocates would cooperate with a regulation restricting its use to the "terminal". Judge Clark states:
"In studied defiance of current law, Dr. Privitera prescribed
and administered the drug as a cancer cure, advised his
patients to discontinue conventional treatment, and warned
them not to let their regular physicians know they were
taking Laetrile."

Doctor Privitera applied for a Writ of Certiorari to the
United States Supreme Court on June 12, 1979 (51).

Legal Implication for Cancer Patients

The legalization of Laetrile, as it has occurred to
date, is partial legalization. The legalization for the
terminally ill removed barriers to Laetrile's use by state
statute or by court recognition of a patient's right to
freedom of choice as pertains to health procedures.

Cancer victims constitute a minority group in our
society; terminal cancer patients, a smaller minority, and
minors an even smaller minority.

The so-called terminally ill are entitled under the Act
to the assurance that the products they seek to use are
effective not only for cure or treatment, but also for these
other purposes. Further, approval of Laetrile for the terminally ill would pose a substantial threat to those whose
cancer was merely "life-threatening." This very real danger
was noted by Dr. Lewis Thomas at the Laetrile Hearings:

> It is often asserted that since Laetrile
> is not a particularly toxic substance, it
> should be made available to all patients who

wish to use it as a matter of free choice.
There is, however, a very real danger here.
If, for example, children with early leukemia or sarcoma, or women with cancer of the
breast, or young men with Hodgkin's disease,
are persuaded to give Laetrile a trial before doing anything else, the outcome will
almost certainly be death in circumstances
where appropriate therapy could be life-
saving (1).

Also, approval of Laetrile for the terminally ill would give
the appearance of an official imprimatur, and would encourage use of the drug by patients who could be helped by legitimate therapy. (See the FDA Commissioner's Decision on
Laetrile.) James Harvey Young, a noted medical historian,
testified in that proceeding, on the basis of his study of
past unproven cures that "[p]ermitting Laetrile's use in
terminal cases gives it a credence among the public at large
that will expand its use in early cases, for people will
prefer taking a 'vitamin' to confronting the surgeon's
knife" (8, p. 39805). Dr. Samuel G. Klagsbrun, a psychiatrist who works with cancer patients at St. Luke's Hospital
in New York, testified that "[p]ermitting Laetrile to be
used by any population of cancer victims would have the
correlative effect of creating the misimpression in the
minds of other cancer victims that the drug is, in fact,
safe and effective for a broader population." Also Laetrile
cannot be effectively restricted to a "class" of "terminally
ill" cancer patients. The experience in this country in
regulating other controlled substances available for limited
use, for example cocaine, highlights the impossibility of
restricting Laetrile to "terminally ill" cancer patients,
and preventing broader promotion.

The danger conveyed by the "gloss of effectiveness"
implicit in partial or total legalization is particularly
acute in the case of children with cancer. Children constitute only one percentage of the cancer cases in this
country but cancer represents the most serious threat to
childlife next to accidents. Childhood cancers are also
acknowledged to the category in which the greatest success
in long term remissions and cures have been made. Yet, the
natural desire for parents to avoid the suffering for their
child which is a part of conventional treatment makes this
class a minority which requires protection from the loophole
in the law advanced in the Rutherford appeal court decision.

A child's need for protection is illustrated by a
recent Massachusetts case (52) arising from a physician's

request to have a child committed to the Department of Public
Welfare for the purpose of providing necessary medical care
(chemotherapy) for the treatment of leukemia. The parents
opposed the petition on the grounds that it violated their
constitutional right to choose the medical treatment appropriate for their child. The record before the Massachusetts
court showed that:

> [A]ccording to the experience of the
> medical experts in this case, the effect of
> this type of treatment on the long-term sur-
> vival of leukemic children has been gratifying.
> After one year of treatment, 90% of the child-
> ren are found to be disease free. In the
> second year of treatment, 70% are in a state
> of remission. At the end of the third year
> 65% are still in remission. In the fourth
> year the survival rate curve flattens to show
> a steady survival pattern of approximately 50%.

The parents had taken the child off chemotherapy and sought
alternative treatment methods for the cancer based on diet
but the child had relapsed. The Massachusetts court affirmed the lower court and held that the record supported the
four tenets of the lower court's decision:

> (1) that acute lymphocytic leukemia in children
> is fatal if untreated; (2) that chemotherapy is
> the only available medical treatment offering a
> hope for cure; (3) that the risks of the treat-
> ment are minimal when compared to the consequences
> of allowing the disease to go untreated; and (4)
> that the parents are unwilling to continue the
> child's chemotherapy, regardless of the conse-
> quences. We conclude that these findings were
> supported by the evidence and were sufficient to
> meet the requirements of the care and protection
> statute (52, pp. 25-26).

The concluding statements of the Massachusetts Supreme
Court are particularly significant in demonstrating the
impropriety of the role of doctor/legislator assumed by the
Rutherford appeals court in its partial legalization of
Laetrile and the consequences of the loophole in the law
which that court would create.

If, through a judicial right of privacy or state statute, a physician's choice of drugs is removed from federal
or state control, and left to the affected individual, a
serious question arises in the case of minors. Will parents

be permitted to make therapy choices for their child which
do not hold out a reasonable hope of prolonging life or
curing disease? What mechanism, if any, will call the
offices of the courts and an adversary proceeding into play
to protect the minor? At what age or stage of maturity will
a child be permitted to make independent decisions?

    In past cases, the conflict between parental choice and
a child's treatment has come to the court's attention because
a physician or child welfare officer at the behest of a
physician has brought it there. If parents select a physician committed to therapies which lie outside the mainstream
of cancer treatment and the delivery of these treatments at
facilities congenial to such treatments and if that physician
does not choose to be an arm of the court for the benefit of
the child, will children automatically be subjected to their
parents treatment decisions without regard for their welfare?
These questions assume increasing importance if the gloss of
effectiveness created by partial or total legalization of
the substance Laetrile becomes a reality. They illustrate
the fragile protections available to the minority class of
children with cancers that hold a good hope of potential
cure or, alternatively, a long remission period in which normal family life is possible.

    The recent Massachusetts court order in a case involving
a minor treated with Laetrile and a coroner's report of a
Laetrile patient death attributed to acute cyanide poisoning
both support the emerging profile of Laetrile as a toxic and
dangerous substance.

    The Coroner of Alameda County, California determined
that a female cancer patient who was receiving Laetrile
treatment died of cyanide intoxication. The cyanide levels
in her blood were 3.8 mcg/ml. The deceased's Laetrile
treatment commenced in March of 1978 with a dosage of 9 grms
every day for 30 days, then reduced to 3 grms thrice weekly,
later reduced to twice weekly and she was on the last course
of treatment (once a week injections) when she died. If the
deceased was unable to come in for injections, her instruc-
tions were to take one 1000 mg tablet of Laetrile (53).

    In the case involving the child, Judge Volterra found
that starting in April of 1978, the parents of the child,
unknown to the physicians treating the child and unknown to
the court, administered the following metabolic therapy
daily to the child:

    1 500 mg. Laetrile tablet
    an enzyme enema with a wobe mugos tablet

4500 units of vitamin A
3500 to 4000 mg. of vitamin C
1 mg. of folic acid
650 mg. of calcium lactate
2 tablets of a mineral supplement known as Seroniums

In tests taken October 9, 1978, it was found that "the child was in no danger of acute poisoning (but there was concern) about the possibility of chronic, long-term poisoning." Tests were repeated on November 26, 1978 and in January of 1979 (54).

Further, the court found that: "neither amygdalin alone or the combined metabolic therapy has any curative or ameliorative effect in the treatment of cancer in general or acute lymphocytic leukemia in particular.

[A]ll four of the parents' experts agreed that amygdalin and metabolic therapy have no observable effect in curing acute lymphocytic leukemia. Dr. Contreras said he could make no claim that metabolic therapy has any specific action against leukemic cells. Dr. Manner conceded that the type of localized treatment involved in his experiments is inapposite to the systemic treatment needed to combat nontumorous cancers in humans, and admitted that metabolic therapy has had little success in treating leukemia. According to Dr. Halstead, amygdalin has had relatively poor results in leukemia treatment; according to Dr. Burk, metabolic therapy does not assist at all in the cure of this disease" (54, p.8).

Finally, according to the parents' experts, the court found that much of the supply of Laetrile available in the United States is "contaminated by bacteria and fungi and is of varying and uncertain strength" (54, p. 13). Dr. Halstead, one of the parents' experts, testified that the form of amygdalin manufactured and used by Dr. Contreras - Kemdalin - was unsafe for medical use, due to its unreliable strength and its adverse side effects, including pyrogen reactions (54, p. 25).

Finally, there are strong indications that the affidavit system for procurement of Laetrile and restriction to the terminally ill will not restrict the substance to that class and will make it available to those whose cancers are merely life-threatening and who could be helped by orthodox therapies. One example arose in the case involving a minor treated with chemotherapy under court order discussed above. During a hearing on whether the child was harmed by the addition of Laetrile, massive doses of vitamin A and enzyme enemas, a doctor testifying for the parents stated that he

did not believe that the minor was terminally ill but that
he would execute an affidavit such as that required by the
district court in the case before this court stating that
the minor was terminal in order to permit the child to procure a supply of Laetrile (55).

References and Notes

1. Hearings Before the Subcommittee on Health and Scientific
    Research of the Senate Committee on Human Resources,
    "Evaluation of Information on which the FDA Based Its
    Decision to Ban the Drug Laetrile From Interstate Com-
    merce," 97th Congress, 1st Session (1977) (hereinafter
    "Laetrile Hearings").
2. United States v. An Article of Drug. Bacto-Unidisk, 394
    U.S. 784, 793-799 (1969); United States v. Dotterweich,
    320 U.S. 277, 280-282 (1943); United States v. Sullivan,
    332 U.S. 689, 697 (1938).
3. 21 U.S.C. SS301, et seq. Originally enacted in 1938, the
    Act was substantially amended in 1962. Drug Amendments
    of 1962, 76 Stat. 780.
4. The Beard Foundation's 1962 application and the circum-
    stances surrounding its rejection are recounted in a
    letter from the FDA files which is in the record of the
    Commissioner's "Decision on the Status of Laetrile,"
    August 5, 1977, FDA Docket No. 77N-0048, 42 Federal
    Register 151, 39768 ("Hereinafter cited "Commissioner's
    Decision" or "FDA Laetrile Proceeding") as Attachment 12
    to AF-15 (Affidavit of W. Sherwood Lawrence, M.D.).
5. Section 201(p) of the Act, 21 U.S.C., Section 321(p).
6. Section 107(c) (4) Pub. L. 87-781.
7. Durovic v. Richardson, 479 F.2d 242 (7th Cir. 1973),
    cert. denied, 414 U.S. 944.
8. D. Kennedy, "Laetrile: Commissioner's Decision on
    Status," Federal Register 42(151), 39768-39806 (1977).
9. Weinberger v. Bentex Pharmaceuticals, 412 U.S. 645
    (1973); Rutherford v. AMA, 379 F.2d 641 (7th Cir. 1967);
    National Ethical Pharmaceutical Ass'n v. Weinberger,
    365 F.Supp. 735 (D.S.C. 1973), aff'd, 503 F.2d 1051
    (4th Cir. 1974); Hanson v. United States, 417 F.Supp.
    30, 37 (D.Minn. 1976).
10. Hanson v. United States, 417 F.Supp. 30 (D.Minn. 1976),
    aff'd, 540 F.2d 947 (8th Cir. 1976).
11. Rutherford v. United States (notes 15, 16, 21 and 26).
12. United States v. Allan Drug Corp., 357 F.2d 713, 718-19
    (10th Cir. 1966), Cert. denied, 385 U.S. 899: United
    States v. 1,048,000 capsules, 347 F.Supp. 768 (S.D.
    Texas, 1972).
13. United States v. Spectro Foods Corp., No. 76-101 (D.N.J.

Jan. 1976), aff'd in part and rev'd in part, 544 F.2d
1175 (3rd Cir. 1976); Hanson v. United States, 417
F.Supp. 30 (D.Minn. 1976), aff'd 540 F.2d 947 (8th Cir.
1976); Gadler v. United States, 425 F.Supp. 244 (D.Minn.
1977); United States v. General Research Labs, 397
F.Supp. 197 (C.D. Cal. 1975); In re Morgan v. Matthews,
No. 76-1637 (D.S.C., Nov. 30, 1976).

14. Millet Pit and Seed Co. v. United States, 436 F.Supp.
84 (E.D. Tenn. 1977), appeal pending sub nom. United
States v. An article of food and drug (6th Cir. No.
78-1202).

15. Rutherford v. United States, 399 F.Supp. 1208 (W.D.
Okla. 1975), remanded for administrative proceedings
542 F.2d 1137 (10th Cir. 1976), 429 F.Supp. 506, 438
F.Supp. 1287 (W.D. Okla. 1977), 10th Cir. No. 77-2049
(decided July 10, 1978), petition for a writ of certiorari filed October 10, 1978, S.Ct. No. 78-605.

16. The action was originally instituted by Juanita Stowe,
a cancer patient, and her husband Jimmie Stowe. After
Mrs. Stowe's death, an amended complaint was filed by
two other patients, Glen L. Rutherford and Phyllis S.
Schneider, and Mrs. Schneider's husband, on behalf of
a class composed of cancer victims and their spouses
who are responsible for the costs of treatment. Mrs.
Schneider subsequently died. By order entered April 8,
1977, the district court certified this case as a class
action on behalf of a class composed of terminally ill
cancer patients. Rutherford v. United States, 429
F.Supp. 506, 509 (W.D. Okla. 1977).

17. S. Rep. 74-361, 74th Cong. 1st Sess. (1935); Kordell v.
United States, 335 U.S. 345 (1948) (mixture of minerals,
vitamins and herbs is a drug); United States v. 250
Jars of U.S. Fancy Pure Honey, 218 F.Supp. 208 (E.D.
Mich., (1963), aff'd 344 F.2d 288 (6th Cir. 1965)
(honey sold for therapeutic purposes is a drug); United
States v. 46 Cartons . . . Fairfax Cigarettes, 113
F.Supp. 336 (D.N.J. 1953) (cigarettes accompanied by
leaflets claiming them effective in preventing respira-
tory diseases, common colds, influenza, acute sinusitis
and other diseases held a drug).

18. Rutherford v. United States, 542 F.2d 1137, 1143 (10
Cir. 1976) and Petitioners Appendix at 32, 13a nn3-4,
14a n5. See Ewing v. Mytinger and Casselberry, Inc.
399 U.S. 594 (1949).

19. Tutoki v. Celebreeze, 375 F.2d 105 (7th Cir. 1967).

20. Rutherford v. American Medical Association, 379 F.2d
641 (7th Cir. 1967).

21. Rutherford v. United States, 438 F.Supp. at 1287, 1298.
The court held that the record failed to establish the

details of Laetrile's use from 1906 to 1938 sufficient-
ly to successfully challenge the FDA's denial of this
exemption.

22. Rutherford v. United States, No. 77-2049, slip op. at
    4. (10th Cir. July 10, 1978).

23. This holding is particularly confusing in light of the
    Court's holding that safety and efficacy have no mean-
    ing in the context of the terminally ill.

24. The Act distinguishes between drugs which are safe for
    self-administration and those which are safe only when
    administered by a physician. See, e.g., Section 503(b)
    of the Act, 21 U.S.C. 353(b).

25. Laetrile Administrative Rulemaking Hearing: Oral Argu-
    ment, Docket No. 77N-0048, Food and Drug Administration
    (2 and 3 May, 1977).

26. United States et al. v. Rutherford et al., Supreme
    Court Docket No. 78-605, Opinion of June 18, 1979 (slip
    opinion).

27. See Tables at pp. 65-71 in the brief Amicus Curiae of
    American Cancer Society, Inc., filed on March 8, 1979.
    In Rutherford supra. note 24.

28. California v. Zook, 366 U.S. 725, 729 (1949) citing
    Charleston & Western Carolina Ry. v. Varnville Furniture
    Co., 237 U.S. 597, 604 (1915).

29. See, e.g., 40 Cong. Rec. 1216 (1906) (statement of Sen.
    McCumber, co-sponsor of the bill).

30. Opinion of the Attorney General of Alaska Re: "Laetrile
    Bill," SLA 227 (1976), dated September 16, 1976.

31. House: Enrolled Act No. 1405, amending Indiana Code
    516-8 (May, 1977).

32. Canterbury v. Spence, 464 F.2d 772 (D.C. Cir. 1972)
    cert. denied 409 U.S. 1064 (1972).

33. E.g., Guilmet v. Campbell, 385 Mich. 57, 68; 188 N.W.
    2d 601, 606 (1971).

34. Hundly v. Martinez, 151 W.Va. 877, 158 S.E. 2nd 159
    (1967) (physician represented that patient's eye would
    be fine after cataract operation but in fact the
    patient became blind).

35. The following states qualify distribution: Alaska,
    Alabama, Florida, Illinois, Indiana, Kansas, Maryland,
    Nevada, New Hampshire, New Jersey, North Dakota, South
    Dakota, Texas, Washington.

36. The following legalize manufacture, sales and distribu-
    tion: Arizona, Delaware, Idaho, Louisiana, Oregon.

37. Alaska, Florida, Maryland, North Dakota, South Dakota,
    and Texas.

38. Slack, "Points of View," The Lancet, July 31, 1977, p.
    240.

39. Roe v. Wade, 410 U.S. 113 (1973); Doe v. Bolton, 410

U.S. 179 (1973); Griswold v. Connecticut, 381 U.S. 479 (1965).

40. On January 5, 1978, the California Supreme Court granted a petition for review filed by the State in People v. Privitera, 141 Cal. Rptr., 764 (4th App. Dist.; Nov. 10, 1977). That pending action is denominated People v. Privitera, Supr. Cr. State of California, Docket No. Crim. 20340. Under California Law, the granting of such a petition renders the lower court's decision a nullity and without force, effect or precedential value. See People v. Murphy, 105 Cal. Rptr. 138, 7.13, 503 P. 2d 594 (1972), cert. denied, 414 U.S. 833 (1973). However, since the case focuses on issues which will be emerging in other unproven treatment cases, it is discussed in this article.

41. Privitera, supra, at 770. In commenting upon Justice Brandeis' most valued of rights, that right to be let alone, now Chief Justice Burger in his dissent in Application of President and Directors of Georgetown College, 331 F.2d 1010, stated:

> "nothing in this utterance suggests that Justice Brandeis thought an individual possessed these rights only as to sensible beliefs, valid thoughts, reasonable emotions, or well-founded sensations. I suggest he intended to include a great many foolish, unreasonable, and even absurd ideas which do not conform, such as refusing medical treatment even at great risk."

However, that opinion is a dissent; the majority permitted the life saving transfusion. The court also held that society has a compelling interest in the preservation of life which justifies state intervention contrary to an individual's wishes. In that case the court observed that there were interests of minor children to protect. See also Raleigh Fitkin-Paul Morgan Memorial Hospital v. Anderson, 42 N.J. 421, 201 A.2d 537 (1964), cert. denied, 377 U.S. 985 (1964).

42. Privitera, supra., at 770. "In Erickson v. Dilgard, 252 N.Y. Supp. 2d 705, a New York court sustained the unwilling Jehovah's Witnesses' objection to a needed blood transfusion despite risk of death. The Court there said at page 706:

> '...it is the individual who is the subject of a medical decision who has the final say and that this must necessarily be so in a system of government which gives the greatest possible protection to the individual in the furtherance of his own desires.'

To the contra see John F. Kennedy Memorial Hospital v.
Heston, 58 N.J. 576, 279 F.2d 670 (1971) in which the
court ordered a transfusion to save the life of a 22
year old unmarried accident victim who had refused for
religious reasons.

43. Privitera, supra., at 20, quoting from Aden v. Younger,
57 Cal. App. 3d. 662, 684, 129 Cal. Rptr. 535. See
also Matter of Quinlan, 70 N.J. 10, 355 A.2d 647. See
discussion of informed consent at pp. 18-23 infra.
There are real questions pertaining to whether the
emotional pressures surrounding the promotion of Laetrile permit informed consent by a cancer patient.

44. The quote relied upon by the Rutherford District Court
"That right of privacy includes the privilege of an
individual to plan his own affairs, for 'outside areas
of plainly harmful conduct, every American is left to
shape his own life as he thinks best, do what he pleases,
go where he pleases.'" Kent v. Dulles, 357 U.S. 116,
126. is found in Justice Douglas' discussion of his
second group of freedoms. Kent v. Dulles is a passport/
freedom of movement case.

45. Under the statutory plan, Schedule II drugs have a medically recognized use but have a potential for abuse
while Schedule I drugs have no recognized medical abuse.

46. Whalen v. Roe, 429 U.S. 589, 598-600 and n. 24.

47. People v. Privitera, Crim. 2034, Super. Ct. No. CR-3278,
Supreme Court Opinion of March 15, 1979.

48. See Note 26, slip opinion at p. 11 text and note 13.

49. People v. Privitera, 141 C. Rptr. 764 (4th App. Dist;
Nov. 10, 1977) appeal pending, Calif. Supreme Ct. Docket No. Crim. 20340 decided March 15, 1979 (47).

50. Planned Parenthood v. Danforth, 428 U.S. 52 (1976).

51. James Robert Privitera, Jr., v. The State of California,
Supreme Court Docket No. 78-1850.

52. Custody of a Minor, Supreme Judicial Court No. P-1422,
Mass. Supreme Court, July 10, 1978 affirming the
decision of Superior Court Plymouth Division of April
18, 1978 in Civil Action No. 78-6916.

53. Alameda County Coroner's Report of 2/1/79, On the Matter
of the Death of Jo Anne Etta Pye.

54. Opinion of Judge Volterra, January 22, 1979, Custody of
a Minor, Mass. Superior Court Docket No. 78-6816 pending
appeal, Massachusetts Supreme Court (slip opinion).

55. Custody of a Minor, on January 8, Dr. Ernesto Contreras
testified that the minor does not have terminal cancer.
He also testified that despite the fact that the minor
does not have terminal cancer, he would be willing to
sign a "Bohannon affidavit" attesting that Chad does
have terminal cancer. On January 9, 1979, Dr. Bruce
Halstead of California made the same statement.

Arthur L. Caplan

6. When Liberty Meets Authority: Ethical Aspects of the Laetrile Controversy

Should the Ethical Issues in the Laetrile
Dispute Be Taken Seriously?

It is no accident that many of the arguments concerning the use of laetrile to treat cancer in afflicted individuals have been couched in ethical and moral language. Ethical language has a good deal of authority and power in contemporary American society. The invocation of language concerning 'rights,' 'freedom,' 'coercion' and 'autonomy' is a powerful chip to play in policy debates. Such language seems unassailable and definitive in arguments about controversial matters of public moment. Once someone has claimed 'a right to choose a mode of treatment' or the 'freedom to care for one's body as one sees fit,' there seems to be little ground for further discussion and debate. Ethical language is often used to stake out the limits or boundaries of policy argumentation -- the point beyond which further discussion is pointless.

In addition to this topographical duty, moral terms often serve powerful rhetorical and political purposes. Disputants in policy debates in all areas of American life have been quick to recognize the hortatory and political force of talk about morality and ethics. Recent debates about civil rights for blacks and women, abortion, school desegregation, affirmative action, and nuclear power have all been couched in the language of ethics and morality. Nothing seems to work as effectively to rouse adherents of all persuasions and positions concerning various controversial policy issues to action as a rousing dose of ethics.

The difficulty posed by the rhetorical or political uses of ethical language is that it is not always possible to discern the pivotal ethical arguments and value commitments of those engaged in a controversy amidst all the

verbiage that passes for public debate. Nor is it always
possible to decide whether an argument is raised in a policy
debate as a matter of politics. The decision not to
'dignify that argument with a response' can be a sign that
an argument is weak, incoherent, or logically fallacious.
But, it can also be a sign that an argument phrased in
ethical terminology is being interpreted as a mere smoke
screen -- perhaps to divert attention away from the real
issues in a debate, or, perhaps to disguise what is in
reality a political, religious, or empirical belief.

    All of these problems of interpretation and legitimacy
surround the assessment of the ethical issues involved in the
use and regulation of laetrile. It is not always clear
which ethically grounded claims are mere rhetoric and which
represent real, reasoned value differences among individuals.
The situation is made more complex by the fact that ethical
language is used by proponents and critics of laetrile to
delineate the scope and boundaries of the issues open to
debate concerning laetrile. This topographical use of ethical terminology in arguments about laetrile has the consequence that the focus of ethical argumentation is constantly
shifting as the parties to the debate attempt to maneuver
argumentation toward issues more favorable to their goals.
It is not a particularly easy task to try and decide which
ethical issues are central in talking about laetrile when
the priorities and weights assigned to various ethical issues
are so open to the pulls and tugs of the disputants (1).

    The delineation of the central or 'real' issues which
characterize disputes about laetrile is made even harder by
the fact that laetrile has served as a rallying point for
disputing camps concerning matters of ethics and political
theory that have nothing to do with the pecularities of the
use of laetrile to treat cancer victims. Laetrile is at the
tip of a very large iceberg of difficult questions concerning the appropriate role of government in interfering for
any reason whatsoever with the lifestyles and liberties of
individual citizens. The nature of governmental authority,
the expertise of governmental and professional groups, the
legitimacy of governmental sanctions, penalties and rules --
are all issues of long standing concern for ethics (2).
Unfortunately, most of the debates about these complex
issues have taken place within the context of pressing policy
issues such as the controversy over laetrile; contexts in
which the half-life of abstract but nonetheless important
issues regarding the nature of democracy, political authority, and scientific methodology is very, very short.

    The fact is that there are actually two main types of

ethical issues that swirl around the use of laetrile. One
set of issues concerns general policy issues about the appropriateness of government control and regulation of individual
behavior and activity. The other set of issues concerns
ethical arguments unique or particular to the use of laetrile
as a drug to palliate or cure cancer. While the former set
of issues constitutes the heart of distinctively ethical disagreements about laetrile, the latter type of issues tend to
dominate the rhetoric and pamphleteering of the actual debate about laetrile. Much more has been written by those
active in the laetrile controversy about the correct chemical
composition of laetrile and the adequacy of clinical trials
of this substance than has been written about the proper
role of government in regulating pharmaceuticals or policing
the medical marketplace (3). Indeed, the only way of dis-
secting substantive matters of ethics from mere rhetoric
regarding laetrile may be to inquire into the general set of
moral issues raised by laetrile use and then to use this
moral taxonomy to assess the actual moral claims concerning
laetrile that are specific to this controversy.

One final general comment about the ethical issues involved in the laetrile debate deserves mention. It might
be argued that any attempt to assess the ethical claims made
in the context of arguments about laetrile is doomed to
irrelevancy at the outset since these kinds of considerations
are not (and perhaps never are) likely to be determinative
of the outcome of the debate. Law, politics, economics,
luck, and emotion are all more plausible candidates to serve
as explanatory variables regarding the course of the laetrile
controversy than are ethical concerns. Debates about scientific or medical matters may begin over ethical disagreements, but, money, power and chance eventually take over
center stage in understanding and explaining the course of
such controversies (4).

The difficulty with this sort of worry about taking
ethics seriously in controversies in science is that when
taken to extremes it leads to the conclusion that reasoned
argument plays no role at all in arguments about policy
issues involving science and medicine. The fact is that
while the ethical proclamations of various parties to the
laetrile debate may fall on a wide variety of deaf ears,
the disputants still feel motivated and obligated to engage
in this particular variant of debate. And there is no
reason to dismiss the fruits of their moral labors out of
hand. Ethical arguments may not be the best vehicle for
understanding the course of a scientific or policy controversy. But they are certainly important elements within
controversies such as the laetrile debate. Thus, their

evolution and resolution ought to occupy the minds of those
attempting to assess such controversies even if they are not
always foremost in the minds of disputants involved in the
actual give and take of controversy.

Who Needs Government Regulations?

One of the key issues raised by the laetrile dispute is
the issue of the legitimacy of governmental regulations of
the behavior of ordinary citizens. The specific issue concerns the moral legitimacy of allowing governmental officials
or representatives to decide for individuals what drugs they
will be able to buy, from whom, why, when they will use them,
and, what they will be told about them. There are a host of
ethical problems involved in this area of governmental
authority and regulation. However, in large measure, many of
these issues are directly contingent upon our understanding
of the nature of the individuals involved as the subjects or
beneficiaries of regulations.

Laetrile proponents tend to depict the consumers of
laetrile as independent, autonomous, tough-minded agents who
choose, on the basis of their values and interests, to use
laetrile for the treatment or prophylaxis of cancer (5).
Critics of laetrile tend to depict these same consumers as
hapless pawns just waiting to be tricked, duped, and deceived
at a time of grave emotional turmoil by money-hungry quacks
and charlatans (6). One need not be a devotee of the view
that the truth lies at the mean to recognize that such pol-
arized views are unlikely to lead to a consensus about the
legitimacy of regulating the sale and use of laetrile.

One way of beginning to get a handle on the appropriateness of these characterizations of citizen consumers of
medical expertise and pharmaceutical paraphernalia is to see
whether certain classes of people might reasonably be excluded from one polar characterization or the other. For
example, even the most vociferous proponent of the autonomous agent model of medical consumerism would be forced to
admit that fetuses, infants, the retarded, the comatose, and
children up to a certain age (say sixteen) are not the
strongest contenders for classification as independent,
autonomous agents.

What is interesting about this group is that the number
of individuals in it is not small, and, that the members of
this group have a number of things in common. They are, as
a class of people, especially dependent upon others for their
existence and survival. They do not have or may have lost
their full capacities and powers to function optimally as

rational agents. They lack the ability to indicate and protect their interests (7). That is, they cannot always say
what they want or need and, even if they can, they have only
the vaguest idea of how to go about getting what it is they
want or need.

If we look to these traits it is not hard to think of
other categories of people who might swell the ranks of the
likely non-autonomous even further. The insane, the seriously ill, the senile, some of the illiterate, some of the
alien or newly emigrated, some of the handicapped, some of
the drug-addicted, and, some of the institutionalized are
all prima facie candidates. This means that the percentage
of the general population likely to be excluded from the
proposed anti-regulation census of autonomous agents is
quite probably larger than those included in such a group.
And this result is obtained without even trying very hard,
i.e., no ideologues, milquetoasts, sloths, sluggards, or
compulsives have been included.

The question then arises as to whether anyone can satisfy the minimal requirements of agency requisite for the kind
of autonomy and independence laetrile proponents have in
mind. This brings us to a consideration of the portrait
drawn by proponents of regulation and protectionism regarding medical consumers.

Much is made in this portrait of the fact that persons
who believe or have been told they have cancer (or other
serious illnesses) are paralyzed by fear. A fear issuing
from both the knowledge of the disease and its dreaded prognosis, and, the knowledge of the pain and cost of the standard treatments for serious disease. The fear, anxiety, and
loss of hope surrounding the cancer victim are presented as
being totally incapacitating -- the patient is too emotionally disturbed to think straight, and is rendered irrational
by the trauma of the diagnosis of cancer (8).

Moreover, persons who believe themselves to be seriously
ill are depicted by the anti-laetrile standard bearers as
particularly vulnerable to manipulation and propaganda.
Desperate people are likely to grasp at any straw of hope,
even if the straw is as flimsy as treating cancer with apricot pit extract. On this view the only way of explaining
the appeal of laetrile among many persons is by dismissing
their behavior as mindless, irrational or desperate. The
choice of laetrile therapy becomes sufficient evidence for
classifying an individual as emotionally incapacitated or
brain-washed.

The difficulty with this picture of the medical consumer
as 'vulnerable' agent is that it runs the risk of assigning
all persons to the class of vulnerable medical consumers in
need of regulation and protection. It is no doubt true that
many persons are traumatized to the point of complete mental
paralysis by a diagnosis of cancer. It is also true that
many people, ignorant of science and pharmacology, will
choose to use laetrile as a therapy in desperation. But,
since there are many trying emotional circumstances in every-
day life that can traumatize people and lead them to acts of
desperation, these facts would not appear to be sufficient
for declaring an individual incompetent to govern his or her
medical life. The death of a parent or child, the experience
of war, bankruptcy, divorce, unemployment and other awful
experiences too numerous to list can traumatize even the
sturdiest souls. Yet, our society seems to feel no moral
obligation to legislate special governmental protection and
medical regulations for people confronted with these emotionally trying experiences. This is due to the fact that
the 'picture' of the cancer victim is conceptually muddled.

The attempt to portray all cancer victims as vulnerable
and incapacitated runs afoul of two conceptual confusions.
While it is true that people are rendered incompetent by a
variety of experiences, it is also true that most people are
able to adapt and accomodate themselves to the most trauma-
tizing of experiences. Vulnerability and incompetence can
be either transient or permanent states (9). If a person
is permanently vulnerable or incapacitated (i.e. retarded,
senile) legislation seems appropriate as a possible protective measure for many types of activities including health
care. But transient vulnerability is an entirely different
matter. It is harder to assess, difficult to endure, and
impossible to prevent. Some cancer victims may be rendered
permanently vulnerable and defenseless by their disease and
their fears. But others, and my guess is that this is the
majority of patients, are traumatized for shorter times.
The only way this sort of vulnerability could be assuaged
at a governmental level is through legislation. But this
would pose both impossible problems of classification, and
swell the ranks of the vulnerable beyond reason since, as
was noted above, cancer is not the only nor even the most
powerful cause of vulnerability.

That government should protect through law, rule, and
sanction the weak, the vulnerable, the incapacitated and the
traumatized is a political obligation whose standing seems
secure (10). But, given the reality of human experience and
human adaptability, a certain amount of vulnerability, weakness, trauma, and incapacity is the lot of us all. It is

the degree and the transience of these states that must be
used to legitimate government concern and intervention.

It is not sufficient grounds for intervening in peoples'
lives to say that they are incapacitated. Nor is it sufficient, as many laetrile critics seem to think, to say that
a person is ignorant. Ignorance may be relevant to deciding
whether a person is an ignoramus about a particular subject,
field, or discipline, but it is not a sufficient condition
for incompetence. Nor is the use of laetrile sufficient
evidence of ignorance since ignorance is being hypothesized
as the most plausible explanation for the selection of this
chemical therapy. Besides, ignorance is often a reversible
state of mind. This being so, regulation and protectionism
would have to take a drastically different tack from their
present course relative to laetrile if consumer ignorance
were the major reason motivating the anti-laetrile camp.

Where does all this leave us then regarding the issue
of who needs government regulation of laetrile? It should
be obvious that there is a fairly large segment of the population who do need some sort of protection regarding the
sale and use of medications. These individuals will not be
helped by simply making information concerning disease and
medical therapies available. For one reason or another this
significant segment of the population will need scientific
guidance and protection in selecting a therapy for life-
threatening diseases such as cancer.

On the other hand not everyone in society needs the
protection of federal or state government in deciding what
to do about a diagnosis of cancer. Even those persons who
are initially devastated by this dreaded diagnosis may eventually adapt to the reality of their situation and be in a
position to regulate their medical affairs without the benefit of bureaucratic counsel. The anxious and the ignorant
may be manipulable, but since this is true of most people
under all sorts of trying circumstances, the permanence as
well as the severity of disablement must be ascertained in
determining the need for governmental help and advice.

Harm, Paternalism, and Protectionism

The argument has been made that the percentage of individuals in America likely to be in need of help, protection,
or regulation regarding pharmaceuticals in general and medical therapies for cancer in particular is not small, but
is not one hundred percent either. One might then reasonably
ask exactly what are those who are manifestly vulnerable
being protected from? The answers given to this question are

important since, if the harms and risks faced by vulnerable
persons are either small or impossible to ameliorate, the
legitimacy of regulating laetrile, despite the existence of
a vulnerable group, would be greatly weakened.

There would seem to be two types of harms facing those
who choose to use laetrile or other exotic therapies to
treat their diseases. These people may harm themselves or
they may cause harm to others.

There are many ways in which persons may cause harm to
themselves by using laetrile. They may worsen the state of
their disease by delaying standard medical therapies. They
may put themselves at some risk to the toxic side-effects of
the drug. They may risk psychological harm in the disappointment that may result from the failure of the drug to
palliate or cure the disease. And they run the risk of harm-
ing their social and economic security by spending large portions of their financial resources on a dubious therapy.

There are a number of harms that may befall others as a
consequence of laetrile use. Children or dependents may be
denied access to medical care in favor of laetrile therapy.
The confidence of the public in medicine and health care may
be weakened by the bad example set by laetrile users. Medical research on cancer could be slowed by narrowing the pool
of cancer patients available for research. And by delaying
in availing themselves of traditional medical therapies,
cancer patients may increase the social burden of paying for
their medical care when they do finally fall within the pur-
vue of medical science (11).

On one reading both types of harm are significant. The
risks of increased morbidity and mortality, or financial
ruin, of a loss of public confidence in scientific medicine,
posed to a rather large proportion of the general population
are nothing to snicker at. On the other hand, the risks involved are no worse than are encountered in many other areas
of medicine and daily life. Strikingly similar cases could
probably be mounted with little effort against candy, soda
pop, guns, automobiles, bathtubs and lawnmowers -- none of
which seem to have commanded the rapt attention of government in the way laetrile and other pharmaceuticals have.

Nor is the protection against harm to the manifestly
vulnerable rationale strengthened when the grim prospects
awaiting the cancer victim are added to the harm ledger.
The risk of morbidity and mortality among persons afflicted
with various cancers is high regardless of the therapy that
is elected (12). And the efficacy and toxic side-effects of

available medical interventions leave much to be desired.
And the psychological and financial costs of the standard
medical regimens for cancer -- surgery, radiation, chemotherapy -- can be as great as any posed by the use of
laetrile.

The usual justification for restricting the sale of
laetrile is that such a restriction is the public's best
interest. The moral foundation for drug regulation is that
the public needs some assurance of the safety and efficacy
of medicinal drugs. Without such legislative protection
quacks and charlatans would be free to bamboozle a gullible
public into the purchase of all sorts of odd chemicals and
treatments. There is a long and distinguished history of
medical charlantry available for anyone to study who doubts
the scope of human greed and gullibility (13). And one need
only look to contemporary abuses in fields such as weight
control, nutrition, and psychotherapy to see that the phe-
nomena of medical quackery is far from being a thing of the
past.

The typical response of proponents of laetrile to governmental protection is 'thanks but no thanks.' Government
legislation is seen as restrictive of the individual's
right to choose those therapies deemed most useful and efficacious in treating an individual's ailments. The freedom
of choice in all matters of personal behavior, including the
selection of therapies and medical treatments, is taken as a
central value and right of each citizen. Not all proponents
of laetrile want to deregulate the drug in order to profit
from its sale. For many the issue is one of defending personal freedom against the heavy bureaucratic hand of the
state. The cost of that freedom in terms of the pain and
suffering caused by bad choices is seen as far more prefer-
able than the burdens imposed by a heavy-handed government
bureaucracy.

In some ways laetrile is a particularly nasty battle
which represents a preliminary skirmish in a broader social
conflict over the value of personal freedom in contemporary
America. Both sides recognize the slippery slope dangers
lurking about the laetrile debate. Those favoring government regulation of the marketplace see laetrile as a first
step toward returning America to a libertarian caveat emptor
existence. Laetrile's advocates also see the legalization
of laetrile as the first step toward removing governmental
authority from daily life. With so many other issues available as topics for this debate, it is ironic that a rather
harmless drug should wind up being cast in such a pivotal
political role.

Freedom and Paternalism

The arguments for any sort of governmental regulation in the public interest are aimed at countering worries about the loss of free choice by the benefits to be garnered from protection. This involves regulation proponents in arguments which debunk the freedom of choice (14) ('Freedom is of little use when you're dead,' cancer patients are incapable of free choices, no one is free to kill themselves, etc.), while simultaneously defending the legitimacy of various forms of paternalistic governmental interventions in the daily lives of citizens. The issue of regulating the sale and use of drugs for medical purposes is thus metamorphised into a debate about freedom versus paternalism.

Those in favor of regulating the availability of drugs such as laetrile do not particularly care to be labelled as paternalistic. The notion of paternalism, especially governmental paternalism, has very negative connotations in our society. Paternalism is barely tolerated by its traditional subjects -- the poor, the retarded, and children -- so it is difficult if not impossible to see how anyone might reasonably expect fully mature rational adults to accept any sort of paternalistic meddling by government for any reason or purpose (15).

The central philosophical reasons underlying the general distaste for paternalism felt by many persons would seem to be (1) that paternalistic behavior is seen as an unwarranted restriction on the freedom of choice resulting from the interference of one person or group of persons with the behavior of another and (2) that people generally think they are the best judges of what is in their own best interest. No one likes to be told what to do or how to act, and it is certainly true that no one relishes being forced or coerced into behaving in certain specified ways. The awkwardness of the regulator's moral stance is patent; either an argument must be made that what looks like a restriction upon personal freedom, the buying and use of a particular drug, is not, or, that in certain cases paternalism is justified.

Philosophers traditionally approach the question of freedom by drawing a distinction between positive and negative freedom (16). Negative freedom indicates the absence of external coercions, restrictions, or hindrances. Physical force or threats of harm are paradigm examples of external coercion. A person who is under compulsion or coercion cannot be said to be free. But the absence of restrictions or coercions is not sufficient for insuring freedom.

A person must have viable distinct options to pick among, or a variety of courses of action available if freedom is to be meaningful. Positive freedom is meant to capture this aspect of freedom. Without real choices, freedom would simply not exist. A man standing naked in the heart of the Sahara desert may be free from compulsions, coercions, and restraints, but his freedom is, nonetheless, severely limited since his options for choice and action are severely limited.

The problem confronting those who want to argue that the regulation of the sale and use of laetrile does not restrict or abrogate freedom is that it clearly does. Regulation, in the form of legal constraints and trade sanctions, almost always constitutes an obstacle to negative freedom. It is simply silly to deny this fact. But it is also silly to think that negative freedom is sufficient for personal freedom. It is not since options, choices, and alternatives are at least as important as the absence of shackles, threats, and laws. Positive freedom is as important as negative freedom in establishing meaningful personal freedom for any individual.

Regulation is not necessarily incompatible with freedom. It is only when negative freedom is restricted without a proportionate increase in positive freedom that regulation and freedom can properly be seen as antithetical. Regulations or laws which do not increase the options available to citizens or promulgate circumstances under which real choices can be made are in conflict with personal freedom. This would not necessarily mitigate against the institution of such regulations or laws. But no amount of cosmetic argumentation will disguise the incompatibility that exists between such regulations and freedom.

If it is true that freedom of choice is quite compatible with certain types of laws and regulations, it is also not clear that all forms of paternalism necessarily conflict with personal judgments of self-interest. An action undertaken in behalf of another is not indicative of impaired judgement or superior insight on the part of the actor. Some actions are simply done in the interests of others as a consequence of the act being delegated or assigned by one party to another. Paternalism can only occur when an actor has not been authorized or delegated to act in the recipient's behalf.

Many persons who participate in democratic systems delegate all sorts of powers to others to act as their representatives or delegates. Large portions of governmental

activities and policies are not paternalistic simply by dint
of the fact that government acts at the request of its citizens and not necessarily from a desire to benefit them.
When the authority or license to represent a person is with-
drawn from government then there might exist some basis for
concern about unjustified paternalism. But when the legitimacy of representative government goes unchallenged, paternalism becomes a difficult charge to make or to prove.

There are situations in which individuals do not consent
to others acting in their interest or in their behalf. Such
cases are better candidates for being designated as paternalistic. But they are not necessarily unjustified simply
because they are paternalistic. If the decision-making
powers of an individual are impaired, if there is grave risk
of serious and irreversible harm occurring, if the paternalistic act is easily reversible, or if there is no opportunity
to ascertain the desires and aims of the actor at a particular moment, then a paternalistic action might be morally
defensible (17). Children, the insane, and the ignorant can
all be the subject of paternalistic behavior since they fulfill one or all of these general conditions.

If paternalism can be justified in some cases, and if
not all legal regulation is compatible with freedom, what
can be said about the morality of regulating the sale and
use of laetrile? It has already been argued that there
exists a substantial segment of the population who are in
need of government protection and regulation for a variety
of reasons. Positive freedom is not a realistic goal for
many people and paternalistic action in their behalf seems
reasonable and morally appropriate in many cases. However,
for many other individuals in our society positive freedom
is a viable and morally compelling value. Furthermore,
despite their ailments and psychological ups and downs,
these people often do not meet the criteria for legitimating
paternalistic behavior. They are only temporarily impaired
by disease, the harm that awaits them is often unavoidable
under any circumstances, and there is ample opportunity to
discern their judgments and feelings about the effect of
laetrile use on their self-interest. Since it is hard to
see how withholding laetrile from such persons could serve
to maximize their positive freedom in a manner commensurate
with the deleterious effect such action would have on their
negative freedom, it becomes hard to see how the regulation
of the sale, manufacture, and use of laetrile could be
morally justified. Once the conditions and components of
freedom and paternalism are explicated, the moral case for
the anti-regulation proponents of laetrile looks quite
strong. If the arguments about the morality of drug regula-

tion regarding laetrile are confined solely to questions of
freedom, competence, paternalism, and harm, freedom will
undoubtedly win out on moral grounds over authority (18).

Filling in the Gaps in the Laetrile Debate

At the beginning of this essay it was suggested that a
general discussion about the moral issues involved in regulation and free choice might shed some light upon the
laetrile controversy. When this analysis is conducted it
turns out that, on grounds of freedom, competence, harms,
or paternalism, there is little justification for asking
mature adults to subscribe to a system in which laetrile is
restricted for sale and use. This is an interesting conclusion since it would seem to imply that, if the laetrile
debate is confined simply to these moral issues, regulation
must give way to personal choice and the free market place.
If it is true that laetrile is relatively harmless, that the
knowledge of cancer does not render people automatically
incompetent, that ignorance is an insufficient basis for
restricting freedom, and that medical science cannot, in
most cases, palliate or cure cancer, then regulation will
have to give way as unjustified on grounds of freedom and
paternalism.

Nonetheless, despite the fact that this conclusion
seems to follow from my arguments, I think it may still be
invalid. But this is only because there are other concerns
besides freedom, harm, competence, and paternalism that must
be appended to any discussion of laetrile. Since they are
often omitted from present discussions about regulating
this drug, this paper will conclude by alluding to two of
the more central of these neglected topics.

First, laetrile regulation is only one tiny portion of
the legislation that exists to guide and direct the daily
lives and activities of persons and groups in various
locales. Legislation, if it is to be effective, must be
clear and universal in its intent. By this political
theorists mean that people must be able to understand the
laws and that the laws should not be ad hoc or weighted
with exemptions and ad hominem provisos (19). Legislation
cannot work if each person is a law unto him or herself.

If clarity and universality are vital components of
legal and legislative efficacy then the arguments against
regulating laetrile may founder on these requirements.
Critics of laetrile laws do not argue for the legalization
for manufacture, sale, and use of all drugs and pharmaceuticals. Rather, they argue that an exception should be made

for laetrile. But the argument for exempting or reclassify-
ing laetrile does not hinge on the generic features of the
drug. Proponents of laetrile argue that it is different
because it has a 'special' history, a 'special' chemistry
and 'special' composition. These arguments may make laetrile
unique, but they also make it difficult to exempt from controls and sanctions. There is a slippery slope here down
which many powerful and manifestly harmful drugs could slide
if an exception were made for laetrile simply on the grounds
that it is a unique or special drug (20).

Moreover, the legislation dictating controls over the
sale and use of laetrile is motivated, in part, by a desire
to control deception and fraud in commercial transactions.
It is, admittedly, an empirical question as to what, if
anything, laetrile can do to ameliorate or cure cancer. But
if its curative powers are indeed limited, then laetrile,
like any other item of commerce, falls under government control and authority not as an object of medical interest but
as an item of commercial interest. The moral underpinnings
of regulating laetrile have as much to do with promoting
commerce and discouraging fraud as they do with freedom and
benevolent paternalism.

The arguments for legalizing laetrile for cancer victims
also run into problems with ad hoc legislation on the grounds
that exempting a cancer patient from a law on the grounds of
terminal illness being present looks suspiciously like an
exemption that is indeterminate and specious. Laetrile proponents cannot have it both ways; either cancer victims are
competent or they are not. If they are competent, then the
type of disease they have would not in itself be grounds for
an exemption from legislation including laws concerning
drugs. Persons who are dying need certain special protections under law, but to be persons they require legal
liability as well. And if this means discouraging fraud and
encouraging responsible free trade, then this must be meant
for all persons whether they are dying quickly or slowly, or,
whether they discern their mortality or do not (21).

There is another issue in addition to the limits and
requirements of effective legislation which must be added
into the equation of the laetrile debate. In addition to
freedom, harm, and benevolent paternalism, considerations of
justice directly affect the regulation and control of drugs
and pharmaceuticals.

Laetrile legislation can be seen as an example of broader legislation intended to protect the interests of a minority. There are many examples of laws in our society and

others which are intended to protect or benefit a minority
of citizens rather than a majority. Tax incentives for
businessmen, affirmative action programs, welfare programs
and the voting rights act are all examples of legislation
intended specifically for minorities and not majorities. If
it is possible to establish a category of persons in this or
any other society who are clearly vulnerable persons in the
sense that they cannot actively and responsibly participate
in the free market of commerce, then it may be necessary to
enact legislation to protect or benefit such a group. It
may be the case that a majority of persons do not require
the benefits and protections afforded the minority by the
regulation of drugs and medicinals. But it may also be the
case that the effective protection of the minority can only
be accomplished by burdening the majority with unneeded and
unwanted legislation. Considerations of justice may, in
fact, require that the majority be asked to suffer in order
to assure the protection or benefit of a minority (22).
This is especially so when the minority is at a particularly
significant risk relative to the majority. The least well
off in any society may have special needs and problems that
demand unfair or unwanted legislative treatment of a majority.

One example where justice may result in the advancement
of minority interests over majority concerns is the area of
gun control. Most people may be able to deal competently
and safely with guns. But there is a significant minority
of the population who, for one reason or another, lack such
competence. Thus gun control may be needed not to benefit
society as a whole, nor to protect the best interests of the
majority, but to protect and benefit a minority. The majority may not need gun control laws, but the minority, due to
their vulnerability, may require them. Efficacy and justice
can combine to produce moral grounds for legislation which
the majority finds distasteful and even coercive.

It is difficult to state in the abstract the conditions
under which a desire to benefit the least well off might
morally legitimate infringing the rights and freedoms of the
majority. My point is to simply note that this situation
can arise and that it may be relevant to the moral arguments
concerning drug regulation in general and laetrile laws in
particular. The retarded, the senile, children, and the
insane may require special protections from fraud and harm
relative to the sale and use of any drug. Most citizens do
not fall into one of these categories and do not, therefore,
require such protection. But many people do and, if they
are to be protected efficaciously and benefitted maximally,
then this may entail broad legislative measures which sacri-
fice majoritarian rights for minority benefit.

It may be that laetrile legislation is paternalistic.
It may also be true that laetrile regulation restricts negative freedom without any gain in positive freedom. But it
does not have to be the case that the persons affected by
this regulation are affected in the same way. The paternalism may only be extended toward the minority who clearly need
it. The infringement of freedom may only befall a majority
who could certainly do without this infringement. But justice and efficacy may dictate this disproportionate allotment
of benefit and burden. Whether it does or does not can only
be ascertained by correctly discerning the complexities involved in the moral arena of government regulation and personal freedom.

Notes

1. Robert F. Rich, "The Political Implications of Laetrile:
    Who Gets What, When and How," in G. Markle and J.
    Petersen, eds., Politics, Science and Cancer: The
    Laetrile Phenomenon, (Boulder: Westview), 1980.
2. Two excellent source books containing extensive histor-
    ical material are: R. E. Flathman, ed., Concepts in
    Social and Political Philosophy (New York: Macmillan),
    1973, and T. Schwartz, ed., Freedom and Authority,
    (Encino, California: Dickenson), 1973.
3. Nicholas Wade, "Laetrile at Sloan-Kettering: A Question
    of Ambiguity," Science, 198, (1977), pp. 1231-1234.
    Also, J. Trux, "New Controversy Surrounds Black Market
    Cancer Drug," New Scientist, 71, (1976), pp. 132-134.
4. Jean-Jacques Salomon, "Crisis of Science, Crisis of
    Society," Science and Public Policy, (October 1977),
    pp. 414-433. Also, D. Nelkin, "Science, Technology and
    Political Conflict: Analyzing the Issues," in D. Nelkin,
    ed., Controversy: Politics of Technical Decisions,
    (Beverly Hills: Sage), 1979.
5. G. E. Markle, J. C. Petersen and M. O. Wagenfeld, "Notes
    from the Cancer Underground: Participation in the
    Laetrile Movement," Social Science and Medicine, 12,
    (1978), pp. 31-37. B. A. Brody, "Quasi-Libertarianism
    and the Laetrile Controversy," ms., 1979.
6. "Laetrile: Commissioner's Decision on Status," Federal
    Register, 42, 151, (August 5, 1977), pp. 39797-39800.
7. For discussions of the concept of interest and moral
    standing, see Joel Feinberg, "Is There a Right to be
    Born?" in J. Rachels, ed., Understanding Moral Philoso-
    phy, (Encino, California: Dickenson), 1976, pp. 346-358;
    R. Macklin, "Moral Concerns and Appeals to Rights and
    Duties," Hastings Center Report, 6, 5, (October 1976),
    pp. 31-39, and A. L. Caplan, "Rights Language and the

Ethical Treatment of Animals," in L. McCullough and J. Morris, eds., Implications of History and Ethics to Medicine, (College Station: Texas A & M Press), 1978.

8. Cf. Susan Sontag, Illness as Metaphor, (New York: Farrar, Straus and Giroux), 1978.

9. See chapter seven, "Mental Illness and Impaired Abilities," in Jonathan Glover, Responsibility, (New York: Humanities Press), 1970, pp. 126-141, and, Charles Fried, Medical Experimentation: Personal Integrity and Social Policy, (New York: American Elsevier), 1974.

10. John Rawls, A Theory of Justice, (Cambridge: Harvard), 1971, chapters one and two. G. Vlastos, "Justice and Equality," in R. B. Brandt, ed., Social Justice, (Englewood Cliffs, N.J.: Prentice-Hall), 1912, pp. 31-72.

11. Op.cit., "Laetrile: Commissioner's Decision on Status," pp. 39802-39805.

12. J. E. Enstrom and D. F. Austin, "Interpreting Cancer Survival Rates," Science, 1975, (1977), pp. 847-851.

13. J. H. Young, The Medical Messiahs, (Princeton: University Press), 1967, J. H. Young, The Toadstool Millionaires, (Princeton: University Press), 1961.

14. Op.cit., "Laetrile: Commissioner's Decision on Status," pp. 39803-39804.

15. R. Nozick, Anarchy, State and Utopia, (New York: Basic Books), 1974, pp. 26-88.

16. G. C. MacCallum, Jr., "Negative and Positive Freedom," The Philosophical Review, 76, (1967), pp. 312-334.

17. B. Gert and C. M. Culver, "Paternalistic Behavior," Philosophy and Public Affairs, (Fall, 1976), pp. 45-57; D. H. Regan, "Justifications for Paternalism" in J. R. Pennock and J. N. Chapman, eds., The Limits of Law, Nomos XV, (New York: N.Y.U. Press), 1974, pp. 201-216; and, Rosemary Carter, "Justifying Paternalism," Canadian Journal of Philosophy, (March, 1977), pp. 133-143.

18. D. B. Moscowitz, "Therapy Choice Increasingly Judged Layman's Domain," Medical World News, (February 20, 1978), p. 80, Richard Landau, ed., Regulating New Drugs, (Chicago: University Press), 1973; and, D. Thompson, "Paternalism in Medicine, Law and Public Policy," ms., 1979.

19. M. D. Bayles, Principles of Legislation, (Detroit: Wayne State University Press), 1978. L. L. Fuller, The Morality of Law, (New Haven: Yale), 1969.

20. J. A. Richardson and P. Griffith, Laetrile Case Histories, (New York: Bantam), 1977; and, M. L. Culbert, Vitamin B-17 - Forbidden Weapon Against Cancer: The Fight for Laetrile, (New Rochelle, N.Y.: Arlington House), 1974.

21. Richard Wasserstrom, "Rights, Human Rights and Racial
     Discrimination," The Journal of Philosophy, 61, (1964),
     pp. 631-650; Peter Singer, "All Animals are Equal,"
     Philosophic Exchange, 1, 5, (Summer 1974), pp. 103-116;
     and James Nickel, "Discrimination and Morally Relevant
     Characteristics," Analysis, 32, (1972), pp. 113-114.
22. William Blackstone, "Reverse Discrimination and Compen-
     satory Justice," Social Theory and Practice, 3 (1975),
     pp. 253-288; Bernard Boxill, "The Morality of Preferen-
     tial Hiring," Philosophy and Public Affairs, 7, (1978),
     pp. 246-68; and A. H. Goldman, Justice and Reverse Dis-
     crimination, (Princeton: University Press), 1979.

7. Social Context of the Laetrile Phenomenon

In recent years Americans have witnessed a tremendous amount of conflict over Laetrile (1,2). Proponents of this purported cancer treatment have battled the Food and Drug Administration, the American Cancer Society, the National Cancer Institute, and other medical authorities in a variety of settings including the media, state legislatures, and the courts. Why has the dispute over Laetrile emerged as a major social controversy in the 1970s? How can we account for the impressive growth of the Laetrile movement during this period? How have the Laetrile proponents been able to achieve political victories in the face of prestigious and powerful opponents?

This chapter will attempt to answer these questions through an examination of the social matrix in which the Laetrile controversy is embedded. In approaching the dispute over Laetrile, we will consider three types of factors: scientific, contextual, and situational. Scientific factors focus on the philosophical and professional variables common to many controversies in medicine. Much of the enmity of the current debate is traced to social and subjective forces within science. Contextual factors include such basic American values as individualism, freedom and equality. Contemporary Laetrile appeals, such as freedom of choice and rejection of expertise, as well as opposing anti-Laetrile arguments, are rooted in such values. Finally, situational variables unique to the 1970s are examined. These include such factors as heightened frustration over the inability to cure cancer, the decline in trust in science and medicine along with the concomitant growth of self-help medicine, and changes in the Laetrile movement itself.

Our approach to the Laetrile phenomenon is guided by Bloor's call for the "strong program" in the sociology of knowledge (3). Bloor contends that the sociology of scienti-

fic knowledge should be causal, impartial, and symmetrical
(4). While sociologists would not want to argue that social
factors are the sole cause of beliefs, they should be concerned with the social conditions producing belief or states
of knowledge. Furthermore, the strong program demands an
approach which is "impartial with respect to truth and fal-
sity, rationality or irrationality, success or failure" (3,
p. 5). Explanations in this approach should be symmetrical;
the same types of cause may explain true and false beliefs.
As Bloor has observed, scholars of science have too frequently sought causes to explain error or deviation while assuming
that logic, rationality, and truth were their own explanation.

For these reasons we take an impartial -- perhaps agnostic -- position on Laetrile. We will not be concerned here
with whether or not Laetrile controls cancer. Further, we
will approach both sides of the Laetrile controversy in a
similar manner. We do this not because we wish to suggest
that both sides have an equal legitimacy, but because an
explanation of the phenomenon should be symmetrical. The
causes of the behavior of both sides of the controversy come
from the same social matrix. Both must be understood to
appreciate the controversy's social and intellectual founda-
tions.

Schattschneider's (5) work on contemporary American
political movements is our theoretical exemplar. Though
Schattschneider outlines a conflict theory of politics, his
work has implications for disputes which are not exclusively
political -- such as the Laetrile controversy. Consistent
with the strong program, his analysis is causal, emphasizing
the role of audience and other resources in the resolution of
conflicts. This focus remains unchanged, though the initial
winners of a conflict may become the eventual losers. Moreover, the analysis is impartial with respect to the truth
claims of both sides. Schattschneider's analysis is also
symmetrical, meaning that both sides of a controversy are
likely to use similar tactics and strategies, depending on
the strength of their initial and developing positions.

Schattschneider asserts that the scope of a conflict
determines its outcome. Disputes are won or lost depending
on the extent to which the audiences are mobilized to participate in the conflict. The main struggle -- and most important strategy -- in politics is over the scope of conflicts.
At any level the likely winners of a conflict will try to
limit the scope of the dispute while potential losers will
work to expand it. As Schattschneider observes, "it follows
that conflicts are frequently won or lost by the success
that the contestants have in getting the audience involved

in the fight or in excluding it, as the case may be" (5, p. 4).

One cannot, then, forecast the outcome of conflicts by simply estimating the strength of the original contestants. The weaker side in a dispute may have great potential strength if it can be aroused. Changes of scope contain a bias since it is highly unlikely that both sides of a dispute will be evenly reinforced as additional combatants enter the arena. Though the losing side generally tries to expand the conflict, there is always a risk in so doing: the new publics involved may be strong enough to wrest control from the original combatants. In mobilization, then, contestants on one or both sides may lose control of the shape of the conflict.

Schattschneider maintained that ideologies which emerge in conflict are best understood as strategic and tactical attempts to manipulate the scope of a dispute. Rather than viewing controversies as value conflicts, Schattschneider viewed political disputes as mediated through the successful appeal to values. Ideas such as individualism, localism, and privacy and economy in government have frequently been used to try to restrict the scope of conflicts, while equality, consistency, justice, liberty, and freedom are often used as means of broadening the scope of disputes.

Bloor and Schattschneider pose a set of strategic and tactical questions for this inquiry: which interest groups have militated for and against Laetrile? What audiences have they attempted to mobilize? Which ideologies have they invoked? And has each side maintained control of its own tactics? In our consideration of the way contextual, scientific and situational factors have shaped the Laetrile controversy, we shall address these questions.

Scientific Factors

Both advocates and opponents of Laetrile have used scientific arguments as tactical and strategic resources in the controversy. Supporters of Laetrile have sought to expand the controversy by attacking the philosophical assumptions of modern medicine and positing an alternate system of holistic medicine. In turn, orthodox medicine has attempted to restrict the controversy in two ways: by attacking the professional credentials and qualifications of Laetrile advocates, and by sponsoring animal studies to show that Laetrile is not efficacious. How each of these tactics and strategies have affected the controversy is considered in this section.

The history of Western medicine can be viewed as a
struggle between the empirical and the naturopathic philosophy of medicine (6). The empirical tradition, from which
modern medicine developed, stresses the mechanistic nature
of the organism and the foreign nature of disease. Viewing
the patient as a complex machine (e.g., the heart as a pump),
the physician treats localized symptoms and repairs or ex-
cises defective parts. Illness is an external imposition on
the patient. Sickness is combated with drugs, and little
emphasis is placed on nutrition. Consistent with this philosophy, orthodox medicine has taken no strong role in shaping
the American diet. There are lip-service appeals to avoid
junk foods and recommendations concerning balanced diets, but
these concerns are generally peripheral to the physicians'
primary work of treating disease. In the empirical tradition
the decisive factor in treatment is the physician himself,
while the role of the patient in treating his or her own disease is down-played.

Opposing the empirical tradition is the naturopathic
philosophy of medicine. Here disease is viewed as "a general
fact which strikes the whole organism and has its origins in
a perturbation of natural harmony" (6, p. XI). Traditional
naturopathy has nearly disappeared in the United States but
two modern versions, holistic medicine and orthomolecular
medicine, are currently receiving considerable attention.
Both emphasize the role of natural substances -- organically
grown foods, vitamins, minerals and herbs -- in the maintenance of health; and the growing popularity of health and
organic foods attests to the vigor and broad popular base of
the movement.

Holistic medicine maintains that

(1) you take responsibility for your own health;
(2) that you see your physical health as part of an
entire life-style, (3) that you choose a doctor who
sees you as a total human being (7, p. 21).

As an alternate philosophy of medicine, holism has made
inroads into, or perhaps has been coopted by, orthodox medicine. Recently, for example, several branches of the
National Institutes of Health sponsored a conference on
"Holistic Health: A Public Policy." In one of the conference courses, "Health Through Nature and Cosmos," a native
American Indian "explores the powers of transformation in
re-establishing a relationship with Mother Earth, The Female
Energy" wherein the student learns "to use touch (vibration),
color, crystals and sound as healing instruments to alleviate
suffering and prevent illness" (8).

Whereas holism seems to reflect popular, or even religious and mystical culture, orthomolecular medicine has its roots in the experimental sciences. Linus Pauling, twice a Nobel Prize winner, has created and organized the new health discipline which he defines as "the preservation of good health and the treatment of disease by varying the concentrations in the human body of substances that are normally present in the body and are required for health" (9). Various researchers have recently claimed success with orthomolecular strategies (10) and articles in the Journal of Orthomolecular Psychiatry purport that schizophrenia can be controlled and reversed by dietary supplements.

The historical roots of the Laetrile movement seem to be distinct from holism or orthomolecular medicine. Nevertheless Laetrile advocates use these contemporary movements as intellectual resources in their battle with orthodox medicine. The most important holistic claim of the movement is that Laetrile is a vitamin, known as B-17, which is necessary for the maintenance of health and prevention of cancer. Absence of Laetrile, according to one advocate, may: "produce headaches, anorexia, bizarre muscular pains, skin changes, anemia, sense of impending doom ... high blood pressure, sickle cell anemia and finally, tumefaction" (11, p. 465). Thus cancer is not a tumor disease; rather it is a metabolic disease in which the tumor is merely an obvious symptom. Just as it takes Vitamin B-12 as well as iron to cure pernicious anemia and proper diet as well as insulin to control diabetes, Laetrile supporters maintain that Vitamin B-17, described by one supporter as the "crown jewel in a total diadem of treatment" (11, p. 353), and diet will prevent or control cancer. In fact, in public speeches Dr. John Richardson, a leading Laetrile proponent, now calls cancer "fulminating avitaminosis."

Even so, and consistent with the holistic view of medicine, cancer is seen as a naturally occuring, degenerative phenomenon. Undetected and undetectable cancer is a part of normal life:

Sub-clinical cancer is developing all the time. It may occur many times in a lifetime. But natural factors in the body itself keep it under control. Only when these natural factors do not keep it under control does the final "gross manifestation," usually characterized by tumefaction, or lumps and bumps, occur (12).

All of these claims are seen as part of a scientific doctrine, and Laetrile advocates claim the prestige of a

science, albeit an officially condemned science. The notion
of vitamin deficiency is seen as part of an elaborate theory
of cancer, known as the trophoblastic or unitarian thesis
(13). Compared with orthodoxy this thesis calls for a different interpretation of cause, of symptoms, of the relationship between theory and practice and of the role of the physician (6, p. XV) -- in short, a different philosophy of
medicine.

Several participants at the 1977 FDA Hearings on
Laetrile recognized the philosophical differences between
holistic and orthodox medicine. According to one opponent:

> ...The Laetrile system is indeed a total medical
> system...with its own biology and biochemistry
> which is different from that of standard science,
> but which is credible enough...that modern day
> sophisticated people will regard it as credible,
> reasonable and something worthwhile to try (11,
> p. 121).

While a Laetrile proponent argues for the concept of
holistic medicine which treats:

> ...the whole man as a single entity, the sum
> of his parts. And once again a light year
> removed from the specialized, fragmented,
> crisis medicine whereby the patient is shuttled
> from dermatologists to internists to gastrolo-
> gists to oncologists to psychiatrists (11, p.
> 352).

The new sensitivity toward, and popularity of, holistic and orthomolecular medicine have certainly served as a
strategic resource to the Laetrile movement. No longer seen
as an isolated product with its own separate history, Laetrile now appeals to many people seeking alternatives to
orthodox therapy. To this strategic thrust medical experts
and authorities have responded with tactics consistent with
the empirical tradition. They maintain that the practice of
medicine is exceedingly complex and can be mastered only by
persons with extensive training. The best guarantee of competent and even life-saving therapy is the professionalized
and highly certified physician. Others, whether well-
meaning or quacks, are clearly acting against the best interest of the patient.

In general the promotion of Laetrile -- and most of
the pro-Laetrile research -- has been carried out by individuals outside the scientific community or by foreign physi-

cians who fall outside the medical certification system of
the United States. For example, Ernst Krebs, Jr., widely
regarded as the major theoretician of the Laetrile movement,
describes himself as a biochemist. However, the FDA has
frequently criticized his credentials. He was expelled from
Hahnemann Medical School but later completed a B.A. at the
University of Illinois. While he is referred to in the movement as 'Dr. Krebs,' his doctorate is an honorary one from
American Christian College in Tulsa, Oklahoma (14).

Similarly the FDA has been critical of Andrew McNaughton,
son of a former President of the United Nations Security Council and one of the earliest financiers of the Laetrile movement (15). Ernesto Contreras, a physician and founder of a
Tijuana clinic which purportedly treats 150 patients per day
with Laetrile, has acknowledged the problem of credentialism:

> Since the beginning, amygdalin (Laetrile) was
> handled in a non-professional way and it was put
> in the hands of general practitioners or chiro-
> practors. This produced an initial prejudice
> from the oncologists and cancer research centers
> (16).

A few of the leaders of the movement do, however, have
strong establishment credentials. For example, among the
advocates of Laetrile are Dr. Dean Burk. At the 1978 meetings of the American Association for the Advancement of
Science he was characterized as someone who had "spent time"
at the National Cancer Institute (17). In fact, until re-
tirement he was head of the cytochemistry section at NCI.
Another scientist who has evaluated Laetrile favorably is
Dr. Kanematsu Sugiura of the Memorial Sloan-Kettering Cancer
Center.

Even so, the FDA claims that few of the researchers
and clinicians active in the movement have any "special
training in oncology or in the evaluation of drug safety or
effectiveness" (18, p. 39785) and that they publish their
results in books and pamphlets rather than in scientific
journals with peer review. The tactics of the medical establishment are clear: only specialists operating through
professionally approved channels should have the ear of the
scientific community. Lack of qualification or evasion of
procedure severely damages the credibility of the antagonist.

From this point of view only highly qualified scientists are capable of making decisions about cancer diagnosis
and therapy. Such a decision on Laetrile was rendered 25
years ago. In 1953 the California Medical Association con-

cluded that "no satisfactory evidence has been produced to indicate any significant cytotoxic effect of Laetrile on the cancer cell" (19). And in 1973, NCI concluded that Laetrile showed no efficacy against a variety of tumor systems in mice (20).

The debate, according to the cannons of empirical medicine, should have ended at this point. Research procedures are based on logical and mechanistic hierarchies; clinical testing is reserved for drugs which show promise in non-human screening systems. Even so, Laetrile proponents pressed for clinical trials. Medical authorities countered that Laetrile was given a fair chance but failed in the laboratory. Based on research done between 1969 and 1973 the National Cancer Institute concluded that it "certainly has not ignored Laetrile. After extensive study, there is, in our view no sound basis for recommending clinical trials" (21).

Since that time the Laetrile movement has become highly politicized, and the pressure for clinical trials has continued to mount. During the same time period the medical establishment has been adamant in its opposition to Laetrile therapy. Nevertheless, throughout the mid 1970s the NCI sponsored laboratory research on Laetrile at Arthur D. Little, Inc.; the Southern Research Institute; Washington University; the Battelle Memorial Institute and Sloan-Kettering Memorial Cancer Center (22). In each of these studies, and to the surprise of no one, Laetrile was found to be inactive against various types of tumors in mice.

We view laboratory studies as another strategic and tactical resource to control the Laetrile controversy. As the pressure for clinical testing and legalization of Laetrile increased, establishment scientists turned to the milieu that they knew best -- the laboratory. Here training and skill could be applied to confirm researchers' suspicions that Laetrile had no efficacy. Here evidence could be gathered for use in other settings -- legislatures, courts and regulatory agencies. And here, the medical establishment hoped, the controversy could be restricted to the logic and method of empirical science.

Laetrile advocates have attacked the animal studies both theoretically, from a holistic position, and methodologically, from an empirical stance. Seen from the holistic position, mouse studies make little sense. Mice take no responsibility for their own health and presumably do not see health as a spiritual issue. Moreover they cannot report the more subjective aspects of experimentation such as the alleviation of pain. Furthermore, mouse tumor systems, whether spontaneous or transplanted, are not identical to the naturally occurring cancers of human beings.

Every mouse study has also been attacked on methodological grounds. The appropriate strain of mice, the choice of tumor system and the assessment of efficacy -- in other words, all of the ambiguities of any experimental design -- have been examined at length in the Laetrile literature. In fact, the Sloan-Kettering experiments came under criticism not only from anti-establishment groups such as Second Opinion (23) but also from the official publication of the New York Academy of Sciences (24).

Laetrile advocates have not conceded the experimental domain to the scientific establishment. Rather, their empirical counter-attacks have confused an already incredibly complex debate. As the esoterica of mouse studies is publicly debated, experimental data of any sort takes on a certain amount of legitimacy. In 1977 a Loyola biologist purported that Laetrile, as part of a megavitamin regimen, effectively controlled mammary tumors in mice (25). Despite the fact that the paper was first read in a non-scholarly setting, that the paper was only two pages long, and that the experimental design lacked certain controls, the paper received national media attention. Now at last Laetrile advocates had their own mouse studies to use as a tactical resource.

Contextual Factors

In 1977 approximately 310,000 Americans died of cancer. In the U.S. in the 1970s there will be an estimated 3.5 million cancer deaths, 6.5 million new cancer cases and more than 10 million people under medical care for cancer. Once cancer is contracted, the death rate is fearfully high. Of the 700,000 people who were diagnosed as having cancer in 1977, only about one-third are expected to be alive by 1982; and many additional thousands presumably will die of their cancers in the years thereafter. If present rates are maintained, some 54 million Americans now living, or one in every four, will eventually die of cancer (26).

Over the years cancer will strike in approximately two of three families. Thus, few Americans will avoid watching the death of a friend or family member by cancer. Given the debilitating nature of the disease and the severe nature of its treatment, cancer may be a disease with a unique social, as well as clinical, character. Cancer is by far

the most feared of illnesses (27). Just as tuberculosis
used to be associated with a romantic metaphor, according
to Susan Sontag, cancer has now come to mean repression,
violence and death (28). Against this backdrop one promi-
nent physician has characterized the fear of cancer as
cancerophobia, "a disease as serious to society as cancer is
to the individual -- and morally more devastating" (29).

One way of viewing the Laetrile phenomenon is that it
is a response to the clinical and social nature of cancer.
In fact, both sides of the controversy seem to agree on this
causal sequence. However, medical orthodoxy emphasizes an
irrational, even phobic, fear of cancer as the explanatory
intermediate variable:

> the answer lies in the fear that cancer engen-
> ders -- and that proven therapies for cancer
> engender -- and the need of patients and fami-
> lies for hope in a situation where the hope
> offered by the legitimate therapies is often
> modest (18, p. 39797).

Laetrile advocates, on the other hand, see the movement's
popularity as a scientific response to the "cancer epidemic."
As an alternative to surgery, irradiation and chemotherapy
("Slashing, burning and poisoning"), believers are offered
a simple and painless way to prevent or control our most
dread disease.

An accurate causal model of the Laetrile phenomenon
must consider several complex factors. For though Laetrile
is a response to cancer, the pathway is not direct. Among
those variables that intervene are several dominant American
values. By a value we mean:

> those conceptions of desirable states of affairs
> that are utilized in selective conduct of cri-
> teria for preference or choice or as justifications
> for proposed or actual behavior (30, p. 442).

Focusing on values as justifications we do not view the Laetrile controversy as a value conflict per se. Rather it seems
that each side of the controversy has appealed to basic
American values as a means of strengthening a position.
Laetrile advocates have attempted to open and expand the
controversy to new publics by appealing to the values of
freedom and equality; medical orthodoxy, on the other hand,
has tried to close and restrict the debate through an appeal
to the values of expertise and scientific and secular rationality.

Americans have always asserted their freedom in health
issues. They choose their own physicians, but they also
choose tremendous quantities of non-prescription drugs to
treat everything from common colds to declining sex appeal
to some rather serious diseases (31). Some also assert
their right to attempt cancer prophylaxis and treatment.
Laetrile, they claim, is non-toxic (32). Yet the Federal
Government bans its interstate sale. From the advocates
point of view this ban makes little sense, especially in
light of the legal status of known carcinogens such as
tobacco and saccharin. Even if Laetrile were not efficacious, they argue, neither are many of the non-prescription
drugs sold in such huge quantities throughout the United
States. This so-called freedom of choice theme is the most
powerful and strategically successful appeal of the Laetrile
movement. It is also a device for expanding the scope of
the conflict. In fact, the demand for freedom has served
as a bridge between the Laetrile movement and both the holistic medicine movement and the radical right -- especially
the John Birch Society.

The appeal to freedom, and against arbitrary control,
is depicted as a constitutional as well as a personal issue.
On this issue alone, many writers, though not endorsing
Laetrile as therapy, have sided with the aims of the movement. As one physician, writing a letter to a professional
journal, stated:

> I hold no brief for Laetrile, but I do insist
> that a sane person has the constitutional right
> to treat himself in any manner he chooses, re-
> gardless of what you or I or the FDA may say or
> wish (33).

In a similar vein, conservative columnist James J. Kilpatrick
has argued that the real point of Laetrile controversy is
not its efficacy:

> The point is freedom. We loose it by chunks,
> by bits, by grains. Daily we yield more
> authoritarian control to the state and to
> the experts (34).

These arguments, so deeply rooted in the American
experience, must be tactically countered. Medical authorities contend that freedom of choice is a slogan used to promote a cynical and cruel hoax. On constitutional, professional and personal grounds they attack this slogan. At a
constitutional level, the FDA maintains that the act of

forming a government necessitates the exchange of some freedoms in order to gain others. In the Commissioner's view:

> Congress indicated its conclusions that the
> absolute freedom to choose an ineffective
> drug was properly surrendered in exchange
> for the freedom from the danger to each
> person's health and well-being from the sale
> and use of worthless drugs (18, p. 39803).

At the professional level, medical authorities have
tried to restrict the controversy by appealing to an ideology
of elitism and expertise. They emphasize that medical decisions and policies must be made by highly trained experts.
The Acting Director of the National Cancer Institute has
stated the elitist position well:

> The average citizen in this country does
> not have the resources and technical skills
> necessary to select, develop and test materi-
> als for the treatment of disease. Neither
> does he have the background that will enable
> him to make enlightened decisions concerning
> the selection and use of therapeutic agents.
> The selection, development, testing, evalua-
> tion, marketing, prescribing and administration
> of materials for disease treatment is an area in
> which large institutions and skilled professionals
> are uniquely qualified to take the measures neces-
> sary to protect the interests of the public (35).

An elitist position logically leads to government control:
those who are expert should not only advise but protect. At
the Kansas City Laetrile hearings a professor of medicine
at the Mayo Clinic asked "Do we want a government which permits the strong to take advantage of the weak, or do we want
a society that protects the consumer?" (11, p. 185).

The strongest attack against the freedom of choice
slogan is at the personal level. The FDA claims that cancer
victims and their families let emotion, rather than intellect, lead them to uninformed choice. As one expert asserted, "the emotional trauma of a cancer diagnosis severely
impairs the patients' and families' ability to engage in
rational decision-making" (18, p. 39804). Others, in even
stronger language, characterize the patient's irrationality
as childlike. Thus: "The gullible, like children, should
be protected from those who would exploit them" (36). This
theme, comparing Laetrile advocates with children, was

developed at the Kansas City hearings where a psychiatrist
declared that:

> Freedom of choice...is the same argument that
> my seven-year-old daughter tells me, when she
> takes matches and says to me, "Daddy, I am
> grown up enough to use these matches, and don't
> worry. I won't burn myself" (11, p. 62).

This attempt to restrict the Laetrile controversy, as
one restricts the behavior of a child, has produced an angry
and emotional response from advocates. Thus:

> You people in authority consider all the rest
> of us a bunch of dummies... You set yourself
> up as God and Jesus Christ all rolled up into
> one. And we don't have any rights"....Patrick
> Henry said: "Give me liberty, or give me
> death." Glenn Rutherford says "let me choose
> the way I want to die. It is not your prerog-
> ative to tell me how. Only God can do that"
> (11, pp. 308, 315-316).

Medical experts have reserved their strongest criticism not
for the followers, but for the leaders of the Laetrile movement. They claim that Laetrile has not been investigated in
a scientific way -- in short, that it is quackery.

This attack on the movement, appealing to the American
value of "science and secular rationality" (30), is probably
the strongest strategic resource of orthodox medicine. Indeed, from this perspective reason and rationality seem to
be on the wane. The government says that saccharin causes
cancer and people continue to consume it; the government
says that Laetrile does not cure cancer and people continue
to consume it. Other substances, such as Gerovital in
Nevada and DMSO in Oregon, have been legalized despite FDA
opposition.

Summarizing the claims and frustration over this issue,
Lewis Thomas, the President of Sloan-Kettering, has mused
"These are bad times for reason, all around. Suddenly, all
of the major ills are being coped with by acupuncture. If
not acupuncture, it is apricot pits..." (37).

Situational Factors

While scientific and contextual factors are important
in understanding the dynamics of the Laetrile movement, four

more immediate situational factors may help to explain the phenomenal growth of the movement in the 1970s. These situational factors are heightened frustration over the inability to control cancer, a decline of trust in science and medicine, the growth of the medical self-help movement, and changes within the Laetrile movement itself.

For the past 200 years medical scientists have cured one deadly disease after another. From smallpox in the 1790s to polio in the 1950s, determination and dollars led to the prevention and cure of a variety of maladies. By the 1970s the primary target of medical research was cancer. In his 1971 State of the Union address, President Richard M. Nixon declared "war" on cancer and proclaimed:

> The time has come in America when the same kind of concentrated effort that split the atom and took man to the moon should be turned toward conquering this dread disease. Let us make a total commitment to achieve this goal (38).

This commitment to cure cancer, now embodied in the National Cancer Act, led to great optimism (or "over-promising" (39) in the words of the FDA Commissioner) in the professional and lay literature. For example, the American Cancer Society claims that: "Cancer is one of the most curable of the major diseases in this country" (40). Throughout the early 1970s, however, five-year survival rates did not go down; in fact, with a few exceptions, they remained constant (40,41). By the mid 1970s, the National Cancer Act and the bureaucracy which administered it had come under attack (38). J.D. Watson, the Nobel laureate, has assailed the war on cancer as scientifically bankrupt, therapeutically ineffective and wasteful (42). "By comparison with the fight against polio," now asserts the FDA Commissioner, "the war on cancer is a medical Vietnam" (39).

Throughout the cancer establishment there is considerable disagreement over everything from theory to therapy (43). Recent debate has focused on the efficacy of surgery for early breast (44) and prostate (45) cancer, combined radiation therapy for cancer of the bile duct (46) and chemotherapy for a variety of gastrointestinal cancers. In particular the use of 5-fluorouracil for chemotherapy has been sharply criticized: "To insist on 5-FU as standard therapy for advanced gastrointestinal cancer offers precious little to today's patient and is a distinct disservice to tomorrow's patient" (47); or: "with this large mass of evidence, one can only hope that the good judgment of the American physician will dissuade him from treating thousands

of post-operative cancer patients with this toxic drug"
(48).

   Despite these problems, clinical research in chemotherapy, radiation and other traditional modalities continues to be funded at high levels while nutritional and
environmental research on cancer is funded at much lower
levels (49). Finally, even programs for the early detection
of cancer have come under attack with the revelation that
X-ray screening procedures may be carcinogenic (50).

   In the midst of this official disappointment, acrimony
and controversy, the Laetrile movement grew. Pro-Laetrile
magazines often paraphrase cancer statistics and official
disagreements over treatment. As doubt is cast on conventional therapy, with its debility and disfigurement, the
promise of simple and painless treatment and prophylaxis
becomes politically, as well as personally, attractive.

   The past decade has also been a period of declining
trust in the leaders of major institutions. In 1976 Louis
Harris observed that "public confidence in major U.S. institutions is at its lowest point since the Harris Survey began
making such measurements ten years ago" (51). By 1976 only
11 percent of the public had "a great deal of confidence"
in the leaders of the executive branch of government, a drop
of 30 percentage points from the 1966 level (51). In this
environment of distrust, it is no wonder that the pronounce-
ments of the Food and Drug Administration and other government agencies are frequently met with skepticism or dis-
belief. This atmosphere has made it much easier for Laetrile
proponents to convince people that the government is part of
a conspiracy to suppress a new and effective treatment of
cancer.

   The degree of public confidence in medicine and science
continues to be high relative to other institutions. Even
so, there has been a dramatic decline in trust in these
sectors in the past decade. Public confidence in the leaders of science was substantially lower in 1971 than it had
been in 1966. Though confidence levels generally increased
from 1971 to 1974, they have since begun to decline again.
Confidence in medical leaders follows the same pattern --
declining from 1966 to 1972, increasing, and then declining
after 1974 (52). Data from the Gallup Poll (53) reveal that
this decline continued through 1977. By 1977 only 39% of
Americans had a great deal of confidence in medicine even
though in 1966 some 73% of the public had a great deal of
confidence in the leaders of medical institutions (51). In
recent years and especially since 1974, Laetrile advocates

have been able to attack orthodox medicine before an even more receptive audience composed of persons whose level of confidence in medicine was no longer very high.

Associated with this distrust is the development of the medical self-help movement. While self-help is not new, in recent years an amazing variety of organizations have emerged which espouse the self-help approach. Some observers have viewed the self-help movement as a virtual revolution in health care.

> Some people have seen us moving toward a 'self-help society.' Others have hailed self-help as the third revolution in mental health, as fulfilling functions in late-twentieth-century life that were once served by the family, the church and close-knit communities, as a sign of an evolving more democratic society, as a reification of the aspirations of the Founding Fathers, as an indication that we are entering an era of self-determination, as the emerging church of the twenty-first century, and as a great many other things as well (54).

Many self-help organizations are critical of, and sometimes hostile toward, health professionals. The competence and compassion of physicians comes under special scrutiny, probably because of the "personal and social adaptive problems of chronic patients" (55). As the data on public confidence in leaders of major institutions indicate, such attacks on the competence of professionals are not confined to physicians. In fact, the medical self-help movement may be closely linked to a more general social movement by outsiders and consumers (56). This movement has developed partially as a result of the perceived failure of societal institutions "to provide nurturance and social support for the needy, the stigmatized, the socially isolated or nonconformist" (56) and partially as a result of a convergence of theory and practice which has emphasized the importance of involving the client in decision-making about his or her destiny.

Pro-Laetrile organizations show most of the properties which have been cited as being characteristic of self-help organizations and they may be viewed as such by a significant proportion of members. One study (57) of a local chapter of the Cancer Control Society found that two types of meetings were held each month. While one was a general public meeting where information about Laetrile was distributed, the second was aimed at active members and cancer patients. At these meetings testimonials were given, nutritional matters were discussed, and social support was provided.

The journals published by pro-Laetrile organizations also have a strong self-help flavor. All contain a large number of short items that provide information on various cancer therapies. Most of these presentations are quite uncritical and frequently advocate questionable practices, such as fasting, coffee enemas, color therapy, and raw juice therapy. The journals also contain large numbers of news items about legislative or legal victories for Laetrile. The Choice and Cancer Control Journal frequently reprint newspaper stories or editorials about Laetrile.

A common type of article recounts personal victories over cancer with titles such as "How I Controlled Cancer Using the Holistic Approach," "Metabolic Therapy Did It For Him," "Beating Leukemia With Laetrile," and "I Would Have Died If I Hadn't Gone to Mexico." Such testimonials appear to be most frequent in Cancer News Journal and The Choice but also are found in Cancer Control Journal. Testimonials seem to be a ubiquitous feature of self-help groups (58) and the major means by which experiential information is expressed and shared. Although most health professionals reject the utility of such statements (18, p. 39799-39800), testimonials continue to play a major role in the promotion of Laetrile by its supporters.

Other contents with a "self-help flavor" in the Cancer News Journal include discussions of herbal teas, health food recipes, and tips on how to stop smoking. The Cancer Control Journal also contains considerable information on nutrition and has examined the health benefits of raw fruit and vegetable juices. All three journals publish book lists that include works on various cancer therapies, health, nutrition, and vitamins. The Choice contains advertisements on a variety of products including apricot kernels, vitamins and enzymes, juicers and water distillers.

Finally, changes in the Laetrile movement itself occurred during the 1970s, and these may be important factors in explaining the growth and success of the movement. Prior to 1970 the major voluntary organization active in the promotion of Laetrile was the International Association of Cancer Victims and Friends. This organization had been founded in 1963 by Cecile Hoffman, who believed that she had been cured of cancer by Laetrile. Schisms within this organization led to the formation of another major pro-Laetrile group in 1973, the Cancer Control Society. Other groups which have broken off from IACVF include the Foundation for Alternative Cancer Therapies (1975) and the Cancer Federation (1978), both organizations which promote holistic approaches to cancer therapy. In the late seventies the National Health Federation actively began to promote Laetrile through such means as its "Fund to Stop Government Ban on Laetrile" and its newspaper Public Scrutiny.

Perhaps the most important of these organizational developments, however, was the founding of the Committee for Freedom of Choice in Cancer Therapy by Robert Bradford in 1972. The Committee was established to aid in the defense of Dr. John Richardson, who was being tried for using Laetrile in the treatment of cancer. The Committee, which today has about 500 local chapters and about 8,000 paid newsletter subscribers, has been very active in lobbying for pro-Laetrile legislation. In fact, it describes itself as "the nation's major leading advocate of the decriminalization of Laetrile."

Since its founding, the Committee has had ties to the radical right. Richardson was an active member of the John Birch Society, as are virtually all of the present officers of the Committee. The editor of the Committee's journal, Choice, has stated "there are a lot of us Birchers in the Laetrile movement because the John Birch Society has the guts to fight for what it believes in" (59). It seems likely that the slick promotional material, active political lobbying, and effective use of the courts which have characterized the Laetrile movement in the past few years may reflect skills gained by the radical right in earlier campaigns against fluoridation and sex education.

Conclusion

Many medical experts and government officials have been perplexed in the face of the phenomenal growth and success of the Laetrile movement. How could a small band of Laetrile promoters garner so much publicity, gain so much public support, and achieve so many legislative victories?

We maintain that the Laetrile controversy cannot be understood without an examination of its social and intellectual context. Our analysis of the controversy, following Bloor's strong program in the sociology of knowledge, seeks to locate causes of the phenomenon. We delineate three categories of causal factors: scientific, contextual, and situational.

Among the scientific factors that we find relevant are

the new interest in holistic and orthomolecular medicine,
disputes over professional credentials, and ambiguities of
experimental design and data. The primary contextual factor
is fear of cancer, mediated through dominant American values.
Advocates appeal to freedom and equality, while opponents
appeal to expertise and the scientific and secular rationality. Finally, four situational factors -- heightened frustration over the inability to cure cancer, decline of trust
in science and medicine, the growth of the medical self-help
movement, and the organizational development of the movement
-- are useful in explaining the recent growth of the movement. Our analysis is also impartial and symmetrical. For
each of the causal factors we attempt to account for the
behavior of both advocates and opponents of Laetrile. Both
the orthodox and the heterodox arise out of the same social
milieu.

In order to understand the dynamics of the controversy,
we use Schattschneider's work as our exemplar. Thus, we
focus on the strategies and available resources of the contestants. In so doing, we do not imply that an attempt to
control the scope of the conflict is the sole motivation of
the actors in the dispute. Rather we maintain that actions,
however motivated, have real consequences for the scope of
the conflict. Medical experts and authorities have tried
to restrict the appeal and availability of Laetrile through
a series of laboratory studies which cast doubt on the drug's
efficacy. Proponents of Laetrile have countered by expanding the conflict into a broad-based social movement. Laetrile advocates, by involving a wide range of individuals
and organizations, have created the most effective challenge
to medical orthodoxy in American history.

References and Notes

1. J. C. Petersen and G. E. Markle, "The Laetrile Contro-
    versy," in Controversy: Politics of Technical Decisions,
    D. Nelkin, ed. (Sage, Beverly Hills, 1979).
2. _____, "Politics and Science in the Laetrile Contro-
    versy," Social Studies of Science 9, forthcoming,
    (1979).
3. D. Bloor, Knowledge and Social Imagery (Routledge and
    Kegan Paul, London, 1976).
4. Bloor also contends that the strong program should be
    "reflexive." That is: its patterns of explanation must
    be applicable to sociology itself.
5. E. E. Schattschneider, The Semi-Sovereign People (Holt,
    Rinehart and Winston, New York, 1960).
6. H. L. Coulter, Divided Legacy: A History of Schism in
    Medical Thought, Volume 1 (Wehawken Press, Washington,

D.C., 1975).

7. L. Grant, The Holistic Revolution (Ward Richie Press, Pasadena, 1978).

8. East West Academy of Healing Arts, "Holistic Health: A Public Policy," conference program, Washington, D.C., 1978.

9. L. Pauling, Vitamin C and The Common Cold (Bantam Books, New York, 1971), p. 48.

10. R. J. Williams and D. K. Kalita, A Physician's Handbook on Orthomolecular Medicine (Pergamon Press, New York, 1977).

11. Laetrile Administrative Rule Making Hearing: Oral Argument, Docket No. 77N-0048, Food and Drug Administration, (2 and 3 May, 1977).

12. R. W. Bradford, Now That You Have Cancer (Choice Publications, Los Altos, 1977), pp. 5-6. This notion of subclinical cancer is also developed by an eminent French oncologist: "We are dealing with an event that is extremely frequent, habitual, and increasingly probable with the passage of time. In most cases, it is aborted, either because the immunologic police are on the job or because the mutation is too monstrous to survive," L. Israel, Conquering Cancer (Random House, New York, 1978), p. 29.

13. For a discussion of the trophoblastic thesis see M. L. Culbert, Vitamin B-17 -- Forbidden Weapon Against Cancer: The Fight for Laetrile (Arlington House, New Rochelle, 1974).

14. R. Lyons, "The Laetrile Lobby -- How Trustworthy?" Detroit Free Press (10 July 1977), p. 1-B.

15. Newsweek, "Laetrile, Should It Be Banned?" (27 July 1977), pp. 48-56.

16. E. R. Contreras, personal communication (16 February 1976).

17. D. Martin, paper presented before the American Association for the Advancement of Science, February 1978.

18. D. Kennedy, "Laetrile: Commissioner's Decision on Status," Federal Register 42 (151), 39768-39806 (1977).

19. Cancer Commission of the California Medical Association, "The Treatment of Cancer with 'Laetriles'," California Medicine 78, 320-326 (1953).

20. Memorandum on Amygdalin MF (B900540), Public Health Service (12 March 1973).

21. R. J. Avery, Office of Cancer Communication, National Cancer Institute, personal communication (4 March 1976).

22. I. Wodinsky and J. K. Swiniarsky, "Anti-tumor Activity of Amygdalin MF (NSC-15780) as a Single Agent and with Beta-Glucosidase (NSC-128056) on a Spectrum of Transplantable Rodent Tumors," Cancer Chemotherapy Reports 59, 939-950 (1975; W. R. Laster and F. M. Schabel, Jr.,

"Experimental Studies on the Anti-tumor Activity of Amygdalin MF (NSC-15780) Alone and in Combination with Beta-glucosidase (NSC-128056)," Cancer Chemotherapy Reports 59, 951-965 (1975); G. J. Hill, II, T. E. Shine, H. Z. Hill, and C. Miller, "Failure of Amygdalin to Arrest B-16 Melanoma and BW 5147 AKR Leukemia," Cancer Research 36, 2102-2107 (1976); A. A. Ovejera and D. P. Houchens, "Inactivity of DL-Amygdalin Against Human Breast and Colon Tumor Zenographs in Athymic (nude) Mice," Cancer Treatment Reports 62, 576-578 (1978); C. C. Stock, D. S. Martin, K. Sugiura, R. A. Fugman, I. M. Mountain, E. Stockert, F. A. Schmid, and G. S. Tarnow-ski, "Anti-tumor Tests of Amygdalin in Spontaneous Animal Tumor Systems," Journal of Surgical Oncology (1978); C. C. Stock, G. S. Tarnowski, F. A. Schmid, D. J. Hutchinson, and M. S. Teller, "Anti-tumor Tests of Amygdalin in Transplantable Animal Tumor Systems," Journal of Surgical Oncology (1978).

23. See Laetrile at Sloan-Kettering: Second Opinion Special Report (New York, Second Opinion, 1977).

24. R. D. Smith, "The Laetrile Papers," The Sciences 18, 10-13 (1978).

25. H. W. Manner, "The Remission of Tumors with Laetrile," paper presented before the meetings of The National Health Federation, 1978.

26. "Cancer Facts and Figures 1978," American Cancer Society, New York, 1978.

27. "Public Fears Cancer More Than Any Other Disease, Affliction," The Gallup Opinion Index, Report No. 139, 24-25 (1977).

28. S. Sontag, Illness as Metaphor (Farrar, Straus and Giroux, New York, 1977).

29. F. J. Inglefinger, "Cancer! Alarm! Cancer!" New England Journal of Medicine 293, 1319 (1975).

30. R. M. Williams, American Society (Alfred Knopf, New York, 1970).

31. See National Analysts, Inc., A Study of Health Practices and Opinions, conducted for Food and Drug Administration, June, 1972.

32. For a contrary view see J. Richmond, HEW News, P77-30, 9 August 1977.

33. J. G. Bohorfoush, letter to the editor, Chest 70, 407 (1976).

34. J. J. Kilpatrick, "Another Uproar Over the Freedom to Choose," Nation's Business (10 May 1976).

35. "Banning of the Drug Laetrile from Interstate Commerce by the FDA," Subcommittee on Health and Scientific Research of the Committee on Human Resources, United States Senate (U.S. Government Printing Office, Washington, D.C., 12 July 1977).

36. A. A. Checchi, "The Return of the Medicine Man -- The Laetrile Story and Dilemma of State Legislatures," Association of Food and Drug Officials Quarterly Bulletin 42, 94 (1978).

37. Cited in "Victories for Laetrile's Lobby," Time 109, 97 (23 May 1977).

38. R. A. Rettig, Cancer Crusade (Princeton University Press, Princeton, 1977).

39. D. Kennedy, "What Animal Research Says About Cancer," Human Nature (May 1978).

40. Cited in D. S. Greenberg, "A Critical Look at Cancer Coverage," Columbia Journalism Review (January/February 1975).

41. J. E. Enstrom and D. F. Austin, "Interpreting Cancer Survival Rates," Science 195, 847-851 (1977).

42. Cited in D. S. Greenberg, "'Progress' in Cancer Research - Don't Say It Isn't So," New England Journal of Medicine 292, 707-708, 1975.

43. For example see L. Israel, Conquering Cancer (Random House, New York, 1978. For a general discussion of such disagreements, see A. Mazur, "Disputes Between Experts," Minerva 11, 243-262 (1973).

44. H. Atkins, J. L. Hayward, D. J. Klugman, and A. B. Wayte, "Treatment of Early Breast Cancer: A Report After Ten Years of Clinical Trial," British Medical Journal 20, 423-429 (1972).

45. D. P. Byar, "Survival of Patients with Incidentally Found Microscopic Cancer of the Prostrate: Results of a Clinical Trial of Conservative Treatment," Journal of Urology 108, 908-913 (1972).

46. D. A. Ingis and R. G. Farmer, "Adenocarcinoma of the Bile Ducts: Relationship of Anatomic Location to Clinical Features," American Journal of Digestive Diseases 20, 253-261, 1975.

47. C. G. Moertel, A. J. Schutt, R. G. Hahn, and R. J. Reitemeier, "Effects of Patient Selection on Results of Phase II Chemotherapy Trials in Gastrointestinal Cancer," Cancer Chemotherapy Report 58, 257-259.

48. C. G. Moertel, "Fluorouracil as an Adjuvant to Colorectal Cancer Surgery; The Breakthrough That Never Was," Journal of the American Medical Association 236, 195-196.

49. D. S. Greenberg, "Nutrition, Stepchild of the Medical Sciences," Washington Post (23 May 1978).

50. _____, "The Unhappy Lessons of Cancer Politics," Washington Post (1 November 1977).

51. Quoted in E. C. Ladd, Jr., "The Polls: The Question of Confidence," Public Opinion Quarterly 40, 544-547 (1976-1977).

52. A. Mazur, "Public Confidence in Science," Social Studies of Science 7, 123-125 (1977).

53. "Medical Profession Retaining High Degree of Confidence," Gallup Opinion Index, Report No. 140 (March 1977), pp. 14-15.

54. D. Robinson and S. Henry, Self-Help and Health (Martin Robertson, London, 1977), p. 2.

55. G. S. Tracy and Z. Gussow, "Self-Help Health Groups: A Grass-Roots Response to a Need for Services," The Journal of Applied Behavioral Science 12 (1976).

56. A. H. Katz and E. I. Bender, "Self-Help Groups in Western Society: History and Prospects," The Journal of Applied Behavioral Science 12, pp. 265-266 (1976).

57. Y. Vissing, "An Exploratory Analysis of Participation in the Laetrile Movement," unpublished M.A. Thesis, Western Michigan University, 1978.

58. T. Borkman, "Experiential Knowledge: A New Concept for for the Analysis of Self-Help Groups," Social Service Review 50, pp. 445-456 (1976).

59. E. Holles, "Birch Society Members Tied to Smuggling of Illegal Drug," New York Times (1 June 1976), p. 18.

8. Discussion:
Bias in Analysis of the
Laetrile Controversy

Controversies, of course, have at least two opposing
sides, and it is worth looking at the papers in this book
to see if the authors have taken one side or the other in
the Laetrile controversy, and if so, how it has affected
their conclusions. I characterized each paper as pro- or
anti-Laetrile, and then passed these judgements among the
authors to check their perceptions against mine. Three
papers are clearcut. Historian Young and Lawyer Monaco are
easily recognized, and acknowledge themselves, as anti-
Laetrile while sociologists Markle and Petersen have sought
a neutral agnostic position and carried it off in the eyes
of their colleagues. The two remaining papers are harder
to classify. Smith is certainly critical of Sloan-Kettering
but otherwise seems neither for nor against Laetrile, so I
called him neutral. I read an anti-Laetrile bias into Rich's
sympathetic treatment of the Food and Drug Administration
(FDA) and particularly in his view of proponent positions,
which I will take up later. There was agreement here among
all the authors but one, Rich seeing his own paper as
neutral and Smith's as pro-Laetrile. Taken together, the
papers are skewed against Laetrile.

If Laetrile is a fraud, a purposive attempt to peddle
a fake cure, then one can hardly fault an anti-Laetrile bias.
But we do not know if the proponents of Laetrile are any
more fraudulent than the median promoter of many orthodox
cancer remedies, which have severe limits to their efficacy.
If the Krebs are frauds, why did they take the trouble to
refine amygdalin rather than sell some readily available
material, as some Krebiozen promoters sold mineral oil? Why
did McNaughton supply Laetrile to Sloan-Kettering for tests
if he knew it to be worthless? Most recently, why did the
Committee for Freedom of Choice in Cancer Therapy cooperate
with the National Cancer Institute in its retrospective survey of Laetrile patients? These instances are reconcilable

with fraud, but with some difficulty. I think that the readiness of many of us to assume fraud comes from false "either/or" reasoning which says that if a cancer therapist is not orthodox, he must be a quack. There are other options. Laetrilists may be sincere believers in the drug's efficacy, whether or not it is indeed efficacious.

Given reasonable uncertainty about the motives of the Laetrile people, I am particularly concerned with the biases of analysis which come from a presumption of guilt. Therefore, the foci of this discussion will be the papers of Young, Monaco, and Rich, where I perceive an anti-Laetrile slant which seems to affect their conclusions.

Young's interesting history of Laetrile is useful for its broader discussion of other unorthodox cancer cures such as Krebiozen. But the historian, by definition, rarely relies on firsthand information, so he must maintain a healthy skepticism about the veracity of his data, particularly that which comes from distant or biased sources. Young is so completely convinced of Laetrile's quack status that he relaxes these standards. For example, Young supports his claim that Laetrilists exploit the cancer patient's panic by noting, "One physician testifying (to the FDA)...told of a patient who, within a day of having lung cancer diagnosed, received Laetrile advertising in the mail." First, we know that the U.S. mail is simply not that fast, but even if it were, one must suspect that exaggeration might have entered when the patient told that tidbit to his doctor, or when the anti-Laetrile doctor used it to bolster his testimony to the FDA. At another point, Young implies that Ernst Krebs, Jr. made unsubstantiated claims by citing, uncritically, this item, extracted from court testimony: "A widow testified that her (dead) husband, learning that he had lung cancer, (said Krebs told him)...that his chance of recovery (with Laetrile) would be one hundred percent." The court record <u>said</u> the widow <u>said</u> the husband <u>said</u> that Krebs <u>said</u> that. Did Krebs <u>really</u> say that?

The most provocative section of Young's paper is his ten-point profile of health quackery, which he applies to Laetrile. Six of these points seem to me to apply to many of the drugs and therapies which are promoted by completely orthodox sources:

Exploitation of fear.
Promise of painless treatment and good results.
One cause for the disease/one therapy.
Shifts in description and explanation of the therapy.
Reliance on testimonials.
Involvement of great sums of money.

One more--claims of a miraculous scientific breakthrough--
seems common of particularly promising new therapies. I
see no strong suggestion of quackery, or even unorthodoxy,
in any of these seven points. An eighth point, that the
promoter "distorts" the idea of freedom, is so subjective
as to be meaningless. After all, who can say that someone
else's notion of an abstraction like freedom is more or less
distorted than one's own notion of it? What of Young's remaining two points?

One is that the quack cries that there is a conspiracy
on the other side. But orthodox promoters also cry "conspiracy" when they encounter successful opposition. For
example, after numerous communities voted against fluoridation, the public health establishment claimed that the opposition was orchestrated by the Klu Klux Klan and John Birch
Society. Indeed, Young himself seems to sense, among the
Laetrile proponents, a conspiracy to defraud. Perceptions
of conspiracy are surely not limited to quacks.

Young's tenth point about quackery is the "Galileo
ploy"--the quack compares himself to Galileo who was in-
sulted in his own time but exalted by history. I think we
do not lack orthodox physicians who have similar self
images.

In sum, Young has listed ten points which may commonly
occur in cases of health quackery, but I suggest that they
occur in legitimate medicine as well. Young writes as if
organized medicine is pristine, rationalistic and altruistic
without elements of egoism, error, and foolishness. He
assumes too readily that pique, paranoia, or greed are diag-
nostic of quackery, forgetting that members of the American
Medical Association share these foibles. To Young, orthodoxy is righteous and the unorthodox are quacks. Laetrile
is unorthodox, therefore, a fraud. This analysis convinces
only those who share these biases.

Grace Monaco's excellent discussion of legal aspects
was particularly interesting when she summarized Rutherford
v. United States, the case which has been the greatest
judicial victory for the Laetrilists (at least to this writing when it awaits review by the Supreme Court). But I
entered that section of the paper well aware from earlier
sections that Monaco does not like Laetrile, and so I was
skeptical of her flat declaration that the district court
which wrote the initial decision was incorrect. The court
found, contrary to the FDA's claims, that Laetrile qualified
for an exemption from the Food, Drug, and Cosmetic Act under
a 1962 grandfather clause, because it has been commercially

available and generally regarded as safe prior to 1962.
Monaco rejects this decision as improper, contrary to the
evidence, and contrary to accepted principles of law. While
the issue was apparently settled for her at that point, it
was thrown open to me. How could the court have erred?
What were the judge's errors of evidence and law? Unfortunately, we are given no hint of his faulty path, and no
opportunity to agree or disagree that it was indeed a faulty
path. The next we hear about the decision is that it was
appealed and sustained! The appeals court made what Monaco
assures us is another faulty decision, holding that the
Drug Act's requirements to show safety and efficacy do not
apply to a terminally ill cancer patient who wants Laetrile.
To my mind, though not to Monaco's, there is indeed a problem
in applying these requirements to a drug intended for patients known to be at great risk from cancer. If a man's
cancer is not curable, then there is not much meaning in
rating drugs by their efficacy of cure, or at least the
meaning is very different from what it would be if the disease were curable. What is a "safe drug" (or for that
matter, a "harmful drug") for a man who is already on the
verge of death? Physicians routinely administer very dangerous treatments in desperate cases (for example, carcinogenic
radiotherapy for cancer) on the principle that if the patient
is saved, then the risk was justified; and if he is not
saved, then he will not suffer from the treatment. Surely
this is a different calculus than is used to evaluate treatments for benign conditions, where dangerous therapies are
not routinely acceptable.

For all I know, Monaco is completely correct in her
assessment of the decisions in Rutherford v. United States.
However, the value of her paper would be heightened if she
would explain this case to us from the perspective of the
pro-Laetrile side, in the same effective manner in which
she argues the anti-Laetrile viewpoint.

Rich's paper is the most difficult to treat because the
bias I perceive, and the consequences which I assume flow
from that bias, he denies. His view is as valid as mine, so
I present these thoughts simply as an alternative view to
consider.

According to Rich, opponents of Laetrile, particularly
those within the FDA, define the Laetrile issue in two
different ways. In one of these definitions, Laetrile is a
purely scientific matter: Is it safe and effective, as
determined by scientific testing? Opponents also define
Laetrile as a quack cure to be put out of business.

The proponents of Laetrile also define the problem in two ways, according to Rich. To them, the Laetrile issue is primarily one of freedom of choice. "Laetrile is basically a convenient vehicle to help reach a larger and broader set of ends. The freedom of choice issues are at stake and not Laetrile qua Laetrile...This group does not make any particular claims for the efficacy of Laetrile." The proponents also define the problem as one of "big government" intrusion into private matters: "Laetrile is simply an example of a more general trend toward government interference in our lives."

Thus, while Rich characterizes the FDA as directly concerned with Laetrile per se--with its safety and effectiveness and promotion, he portrays the proponents as only incidentally concerned with the drug, using it as a convenient vehicle to promote a different goal: personal freedom from intrusion by big government.

Rich apparently denies that any of the Laetrilists have a sincere concern for the drug's fate, and for the cancer patients who might use it, quite apart from their concerns about government regulation. Even allowing that a portion of the Laetrile promotion may be fraudulent, it seems to me that there is no doubt that some of the proponents believe that the drug is beneficial. Surely a major problem, as defined by these people, is to make Laetrile legally available to cancer victims in the United States. Why else did Glen Rutherford, a cancer patient who used Laetrile himself, bring suit against the FDA to have the sale legalized? (See Young and Monaco for discussions of Rutherford v. United States.) His argument that the drug is exempt from FDA restrictions because of the 1962 grandfather clause of the Food, Drug, and Cosmetics Act, does not establish any general principle upholding freedom from government regulation. It is a specific exclusion for a particular drug: Laetrile. Yet Rich denies that in any important way, the proponents define their problem as one of making a beneficial drug legally marketable. That he grants the FDA the straightforward goal of reacting to the drug on its merits, and then denies the proponents a similar goal, is best explained by his own bias, in my view.

Any analysis of Laetrile must carry some bias; even neutrality is a bias. What, then, is the proper bias here? It seems to me that any bias will do as well, or as poorly, as another. The essential point is that the analyst must recognize his bias, he must recognize how it affects his perception and presentation of evidence, and he must recognize how it predisposes him to one or another conclusion.

He ought to consider how another analyst, coming at the same
data with a different bias, might reach different conclusions. He should consider the degree to which his perceptions and conclusions depend on his particular bias rather
than on "objective fact," and when he has eliminated from
his work any major distortions due to bias, he should inform
the reader of those routine distortions which remain.

9. Discussion:
Science and Technology
in the Pits

> Today's American ideologue is a middle-class man
> who objects to his dependence on science even
> when he accepts its norms. He is resentful of
> the superiority of the educated, and antagonistic
> to knowledge. His ideology...looks back to a
> more bucolic age of individuality and localism,
> in which parochial values of mind were precisely
> those most esteemed, to a simple democracy...
> (David Apter, _Ideology and Discontent_).

The papers in this symposium on the politics of the
Laetrile controversy are linked by a common theme; namely
that the dispute has less to do with the curative power of
apricot pits than with the social and political implications
of expert control over an area of personal health. In this
sense I look at this dispute as but one of a whole series of
controversies over quite different areas of science. Many
different concerns have provoked such controversies: the
fear of risk, the fear that a technology can be put to pernicious use, or that it may threaten traditional values.
But an overwhelming source of conflict is the infringement
of technology on individual rights and on freedom of choice.
Indeed, the Laetrile dispute must be seen in the context of
many other disputes--over the automobile airbag, over swine
flu vaccination, and over FDA bans on saccharin and other
food additives. Above all, the Laetrile dispute resembles
the recent creation-evolution controversy, as creationists
demanded equal time for teaching creation theory in public
schools (1).

In each of these cases, the government has imposed certain regulations or mandated certain practices on the assumption that individual choices have social costs, or that
individuals may fail to make enlightened choices on their
own behalf. And in each case there are striking similarities

in the arguments developed during the controversies as well
as in the dynamics and tactics of disputes. These protests
all reflect a perception that government is intruding un-
necessarily into daily life, and that the authority of expertise is intruding on individual choice. The creationists,
for example, argue that government-organized biology curric-
ula based on evolutionary assumptions violates their religious values. Students should, they claim, hear both sides--
evolution and creation theory--and be free to make their own
choice. "Sound educational practice requires teaching creation as an alternate theory so that students can decide what
to believe for themselves." Those who oppose government
constraints on the use of nitrites or the sale of saccharin
want the freedom to make their own choices about risk. Indeed, they claim to have a constitutional right to maintain
such freedom of choice. Curiously, in the case of the re-
combinant DNA dispute, it is the scientific community faced
with the regulation of research which argues, in very similar terms, about the constitutional basis of freedom of
scientific inquiry and the right to pursue scientific research.

The discourse in the Laetrile dispute that was laid out
by Professor Young is also familiar to those of us who have
studied other conflicts. Like the pro-Laetrile people,
creationists use the "Galileo ploy," arguing that scientists
may criticize us now but will honor us later. They too see
the actions of the scientific establishment as a conspiracy,
suppressing divergent ideas in order to maintain power and
control. The arguments of creationists like those of the
Laetrile group shift with agility to meet changing circumstances. Creationists skillfully maneuver around empirical
data supporting evolutionary principles by accusing biolo-
gists of basing their findings on unproven assumptions--
that is, on faith. Based on circumstantial evidence, they
argue, evolution theory is but "a hallowed religious dogma
that must be defended by censorship of contrary arguments."

Tactically, there are also striking similarities among
these disputes, in particular in their mix of technical
argumentation with appeals to basic values. Appeals to freedom, equity, and justice help to broaden the scope of controversy, attracting wide public sympathy; and engaging in technical debate provides legitimacy. The Laetrile folks have
their own scientific expertise; the creationists call themselves "scientific creationists." Membership in creationist
organizations requires a degree in natural science, although
to be sure their credentials are often of dubious origin, as
in the case of Laetrile's Dr. Krebs. And like the Laetrile
experts, creationists also focus their argument on scienti-

fic issues, attacking what they perceive to be weaknesses in
the scientific base of evolutionary theory. This helps to
support their case in the state textbook commissions and
local school boards. But the basic appeal to their constituency of fundamentalists lies in the perceived threat to
religious values.

Similar tactics appear in the disputes over abortion
and fetal research. Here the arguments revolve around the
technical criteria that define the beginning of life, but
these only provide legitimacy to the moral issues underlying
the dispute. Similarly, those opposing the ban on saccharin
focus on questions about the adequacy of animal tests and
the validity of the FDA experiments.

In each case, taking part in technical arguments is a
means to win legitimacy for views which counter the consensus of the scientific establishment. Indeed, a striking
characteristic of all these debates is the pervasive belief,
expressed in the behavior of the protagonists, that technical
debate has more political credence than the expression of
political and value concerns.

As it turns out, engaging in technical debate is a
skillful tactic, for characteristically the science establishment falls into the trap by overreacting to the challenges to their expertise. Again there are striking similarities in the defensive response of scientists. First, they
argue the necessity of expertise to ensure consumer protection: Cancer patients, children in public schools, automobile drivers are all vulnerable for one reason or another
and not necessarily able to make informed or effective
choices on their own behalf. The broad consensus of the
scientific community--about the necessity of teaching evolution theory or the safety and effectiveness of new drugs--is
seen as more important in such cases than individual freedom
of choice. This argument, of course, reinforces the concern
about professional paternalism.

Second, the scientific community responds characteristically by trying to limit the scope of arguments to the
technical arena. But this seldom distresses the scientific
creationists or pro-Laetrile types. For technical expertise
can be found to support any point of view, and engaging in
technical debate enhances the legitimacy of their arguments.
They need not, after all, provide a full refutation, but
only raise public doubts about the established scientific
view.

Third, scientists in all these disputes dismiss the

opposition by debunking the credentials of their critics;
they are "quacks," they "lack qualifications," or they have
"marginal degrees." This too only exacerbates the debate,
lending credence to the arguments about the closed and arbitrary nature of established expertise and its own vested
interests.

Finally, scientists dismiss their critics for their
political motivations, labeling them right-wing or ultra-
conservative. This indeed seems to be the case in the
Laetrile dispute and also in the creation controversy.
Interestingly, in both cases important support for these
movements comes from engineers and technicians in California's science-based industries. But the resistance to
government authority extends beyond the ultra-conservative
fringe. It is not only the right which opposes the airbag
or the swine flu vaccine in the name of individual freedom.
And certainly those who argue the right of women to seek
abortion cannot be labeled conservative. There is in fact
a strong convergence of liberal and conservative values
pervading most of these disputes. Indeed the controversy
over Laetrile is but one example of widespread ideological
resistance to the rationality and reductionism epitomized
by science, and broad political resistance to the pervasive
influence of professional expertise in many areas of personal
life.

Note

1. See Dorothy Nelkin (ed.), Controversy: Politics of
   Technical Decisions (Sage Publications, Beverly Hills,
   1979); and Dorothy Nelkin, Science Textbook Controversies
   (MIT Press, Cambridge, 1978).

Index

abortion, 183. *See also*
 Roe v. Wade
Alaska, state statutes
 concerning Laetrile,
 9n, 116
Allergenase, 12
Altman, L., 69
American Cancer Society, 5,
 29, 44, 106
American Medical Associ-
 ation, 45, 177
American Medical Liberty
 League, 47
American Weekly, 19
amygdalin, 8n, 107, 115
authority, 145

Bal-Sa-Me-A, Syrup, 12
Beard, J., 12, 14
Bee-Seventeen, 27–28.
 See also vitamin B–17
bias, 175, 179–180
Biozymes International
 Ltd., 18
Bloor, D. 151–152
Bohanon, L., 30–32, 48, 50,
 85
Bradford, R. W., 25–26, 30,
 33–34, 36–38, 43–44,
 47–48, 82, 168
Brandeis, L., 131
Brandreth, B., 42–43
Burk, D., 2, 21–23, 27,
 31, 102, 127, 157

California Board of Medical
 Quality Assurance, 25
California, health/safety
 code, 120
California Medical Association, 15–16, 157
cancer
 in children, 124, 128
  parents rights, 125–126;
  therapy choices, 124–129
 child's need for protection,
  124–129
 image of, 40
 orthodox treatment, 176
 pattern of unorthodoxies,
  38–48
 patients, as minority
  group, 123
 patients, terminal, 108,
  109, 122, 123, 178
  determination of, 109;
  drug safety and, 111;
  exemption from federal
  drug laws, 110–111, 122
 quackery, 39, 119, 121
 remissions, 124–125
 victims, fears of, 120
Cancer Control Society, 2, 4,
 49, 81, 166–167
Cancer Federation, 168
Cassels, D., 69
Catholic Medical Center,
 63
chymotrypsin, 12

Committee for Freedom of
  Choice in Cancer Therapy,
  2, 25–26, 29, 49, 63, 81,
  82, 106, 168, 175
conspiracy theory, 44, 177.
  See also trust
Contreras, E., 22–24, 26,
  30, 36, 46, 127, 132,
  157
controversies, in science,
  135, 136
Culbert, M., 34

Damon Runyon Cancer Fund, 19
Delaney Clause, 83. *See
  also* Laetrile, state
  laws
Douglas, W., 116–118
Durovic brothers, 41–42, 48
Durovic v. Richardson, 128

ethical language, 133, 134
expert control, implications
  of, 181
Eyerly, R., 1

FDA. *See* Food and Drug
  Administration
fear, exploitation of, 41
Food and Drug Administration,
  4, 15, 17–21, 23–24,
  26–34, 39, 44, 46, 48,
  50, 73, 74, 76–77, 82,
  84, 85–86, 91, 93, 157,
  161–162, 165, 175, 178,
  179, 181
  Commissioner of, 77, 79
Food, Drug, and Cosmetic
  Act, 78, 83, 91
  burden of proof, 119
  congressional intent, 111
  grandfather provisions,
    102, 110
    of 1962 Act, 102, 106,
    107, 177, 179; of 1938
    Act, 102, 106, 107
  interstate commerce, 112
  labeling, 107, 119
  legislative history, 110,
    129

new drug, 104, 105
preemption, 112
premarketing requirements,
  103, 119, 121
safety/efficacy, general
  recognition of, 100,
  104, 108, 111
  See also Laetrile, state
  laws
Foundation for Alternative
  Cancer Therapies, 168
Fountain, L. H., 23–24
freedom of choice, 7, 22–26,
  29–30, 31–32, 47, 78, 80,
  94, 141, 142, 145, 161–
  163, 177, 179, 181–182
freedom
  impact of professional
    expertise on individual,
    184
  positive and negative, 142,
    143, 144

Galileo ploy, 44, 177, 182
Gallup Poll, 165
Gerovital, 79
Glyoxilide, 40, 41, 48–49
Good, R., 70
Good Manufacturing Practices,
  89
government
  interference by, 83, 94, 181
  regulations of, 135, 136,
    146, 147
  role of, 134
Griffin, G. E., 2, 34
Griswold v. Connecticut, 130
Gurchot, C., 14

Halstead, B., 127
Harper, H. W., 37–38
Harris Poll, 1, 34, 81–82,
  165
Hart, F., Jr., 16, 22–24, 49
Hartman, S., 43
Harvey, W., 44
health quackery, profile of,
  41–48
Hearings: Kennedy Laetrile
  Hearings of 1977, 100, 123,

124-128. *See also*
Kennedy, E. M.
Hevesi, A. G., 91
Hoffman, C. P. 22, 167
holistic medicine, 153-156,
161, 169
Hoxsey, H., 17, 21, 22-23,
40-44, 44, 46, 48-49
Hoxsey treatment, 79
Hunzakuts, 6

IND. *See* Investigational
New Drug Application
ignorance, 139
Indiana, state statutes
concerning laetrile, 113
Ingelfinger, F. J., 35, 64
informed consent, 113,
114, 115
effect of patient belief,
114
effect of physician
representations/be-
lief, 114-117
International Association
of Cancer Victims and
Friends, 2, 22, 49, 81,
168
Investigational New Drug
Application, 76, 101
Ivy, A., 21, 41, 48

John Beard Memorial Foundation, 14, 18-19, 30,
76, 101, 128
John Birch Society, 2, 25,
33, 63, 161, 168
Johnson's Mild Combination
Treatment for Cancer, 39
Jukes, T. H. 27, 31, 50
justice, 147

Kayden, H., 69
Kefauver, E., 17
Kefauver-Harris amendments,
79. *See also* Laetrile,
state laws
Kennedy, D., 8n, 31-33, 35,
37, 46, 85, 103, 128,
162, 164

Kennedy, E. M., 27, 34-35,
43, 100, 128. *See also*
Hearings
Kittler, G., 15, 19-22
Klagsbrun, S., 109, 124
Koch, W. F., 40, 43-44, 48
Koch treatment, 79
Krebiozen, 21, 41, 44, 48-50,
79, 105, 175, 176
Krebs, B., 24
Krebs, E., Jr., 2, 11, 13-24,
26-27, 36-37, 39, 42-45,
53n, 76, 106, 157, 175,
176
Krebs, E., Sr., 11-14, 16,
20-21, 26, 42-43, 76, 175
Kreb's Research Laboratories,
14, 19

Laetrile
adulteration/misbranding,
113, 119, 127
appetite stimulant, 114
bias for/against, 175
chemical composition, 103
commercially used or sold,
104, 106
conditions of administration
intravenous, 108, 126;
oral, 108, 126
criticism, 15-16, 23, 27,
31-32, 34-35, 45
cyanide poisoning, 108, 126,
127
empirical studies, 158-159
in Europe, 89
explanations of purported
action, 14, 18, 26, 37,
43, 45
FDA rulemaking proceeding,
103, 112, 124, 128, 130
as food, 99, 104, 105
hazards of, 6, 32-33, 127,
140
investigational use, 106
issue, definition of, 178
manufacture, 104
in Mexico, 89
money involved, 47-48

morality of legislation,
144
origin, 12-13
pain relief, 114
promotion, 14, 16-17, 19-
30, 34, 41-49
as quack cure, 79, 175
regulatory action, 17-26,
28-34, 50
as scientific controversy,
77, 175, 182
seizure, 104
state laws, 9n, 28-30, 49-
50, 74, 76, 84-90, 112,
113-116, 123, 125, 130
state statutes
hospital, interference,
116; state boards of
health, 113, 121; doctor/
patient relationship,
115. *See also* Delaney
Clause; Food, Drug, and
Cosmetic Act; Kefauver-
Harris amendments;
individual states
uniqueness of, 146
as vitamin, 99, 104, 124
See also hearings
Laetrile legislation,
appropriateness of, 138,
146
need for, 139
effectiveness, 145
exemptions from 145,
146
for minority protection,
147, 148
Laetrile movement, characterizations of users,
3, 4
autonomous agent model,
136, 137
emotionally incapacitated,
137, 138
vulnerable, 137, 138, 139,
140, 146, 147
Leptinol, Syrup, 1-2
life-threatening illness,
111, 120, 123

malpractice, 115
Manner, H., 35, 127, 159
Martin, D., 63, 69
McDonald, L. P., 33
McNaughton, A. R. L., 17-26,
29, 102, 157, 175
McNaughton Foundation, 18-22,
62-63, 76, 101
medical charlatanry, 141, 176
medicine, philosophy of
Western, 154. *See also*
holistic medicine; natur-
opathy; orthomolecular
medicine
Memorial Sloan-Kettering Cancer
Center, 2, 7, 159, 175
Menninger, Karl, 40
metabolic therapy, 37-38, 43,
126-127
Moertel, C. G., 35
Morales, B. L., 2
Moss, R., 65, 69

National Cancer Institute,
4, 5, 6, 7, 8, 22, 35-38,
44, 46, 50, 61, 73, 158,
175
National Health Federation,
2, 22-23, 27, 49, 81, 168
National League for Medical
Freedom, 47
naturopathy, 154. *See also*
medicine, philosophy of
Western
Nevada, state statutes concern-
ing Laetrile, 115
New York Academy of Sciences,
69, 159
National Cancer Act, 164
Newell, G., 5
Nieper, H., 36
Nixon, R. N., 164

Oklahoma, state statute
concerning Laetrile, 115
Old, L., 62, 66
one cause/one therapeutic
system, 42-43

orthmolecular medicine, 154–156, 169
orthodox treatment profile, 176

painless treatment and good results, promise of, 42
pangamic acid, 2, 12, 19, 37
paternalism, 142, 143, 144, 148, 182, 183
pattern of cancer unorthodoxies, 38–48
Pauling, L., 155
People v. Privitera, 117–122, 130–132
physician liability, 113
physicians' rights, 120
placebo effect, 46
Planned Parenthood v. Danforth, 122, 132
political controversy, 74
Posse Comitatus, 2
Privitera, J. 119
problem definitions, 75–76
public hearings, 88

quackery, 79–80, 175–176
accusations of, 184
profile of, 176, 178
reasons for resurgence, 38–40, 48, 50

regulation, safety and efficacy rationale, 141
effects of, 143
representative government, 143, 144
Reynolds, J. W., 92
Richardson, E., 23–24
Richardson, J. A., 2, 6, 25–27, 33–34, 42–46, 47, 63, 155, 168
Richmond, J., 73
"right to die with dignity," 74
Roe v. Wade, 117, 122, 130
Rutherford, G. L., 8, 30–32, 50, 179
Rutherford v. American Medical Association, 105
Rutherford v. United States
appeals court decision, 108, 110, 122, 123, 124, 125, 129, 178
district court decision, 103, 104, 106, 107, 112, 116, 118, 119, 120, 122, 128, 129, 177
Supreme Court opinion, 110–112, 121, 130

Sarcarcinase, 13
Schattschneider, E. E., 152–153, 169
Schmidt, B., 61
Science for the People, 65
scientific breakthrough, claims of, 42, 176
Second Opinion, 2, 65–66, 159
self-help movement, 166
shifts in position to adjust to circumstances, 44–45
Slack, W., 116
Sloan-Kettering. *See* Memorial Sloan-Kettering Cancer Center
Sontag, S., 40, 47, 160
Spicer-Gerhard Company, 14
state bureau of drugs, 86, 89
Stang, A., 74
statutes. *See* Food, Drug, and Cosmetic Act; *individual states*
Stock, C., 62
Stockert, E., 66–67
Sugiura, K., 62, 157
Symms, S. D., 28

testimonials, 45–46
tetrahydrocannabinol, 93
Thalidomide disaster, 91
Thomas, L., 62, 123, 163
Thompson, J., 86
toxicity, 107, 123, 126
trophoblastic theory, 6, 12, 14–15, 43, 156
trust, of public in authority figures, 165–166
Tutoki v. Celebrezze, 105

United States Constitution
  compelling state interest,
    119
  rational basis text,
    118–119
  refusal of medical treat-
    ment, 117
  right of privacy, 110, 116,
    117, 121, 125
United States Food and Drug
    Administration. *See*
    Food and Drug Administra-
    tion
United States Supreme

Court, 74
Upton, A., 36, 38

vitamin amendments of 1976,
  49
vitamin B-15, 12, 19, 37
vitamin B-17, 8, 26–27, 37,
  43, 49, 155. *See also*
  Laetrile
Volterra, G., 126, 132

Watson, J. D., 164
Whalen v. Roe, 118, 121–122,
  132

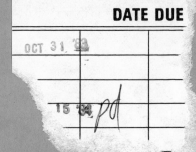